The Memory Prescription

ALSO BY DR. GARY SMALL:

The Memory Bible: An Innovative Strategy for Keeping Your Brain Young

The Memory Prescription

Dr. Gary Small's 14-Day Plan to
Keep Your Brain and Body Young

Gary Small, M.D.
with
Gigi Vorgan

HYPERION New York

Photographs in Chapters 3, 6, and 9 by Rena Small.

Copyright © 2004 Gary Small, M.D.

Library of Congress Cataloging-in-Publication Data

Small, Gary W.
    The memory prescription : Dr. Gary Small's 14-day plan to keep your brain and body young / by Gary Small, with Gigi Vorgan.—1st ed.
        p. cm.
Includes bibliographical references.
ISBN 1-4013-0066-9
    1. Memory—Popular works. 2. Memory disorders—Prevention—Popular works. 3. Physical fitness. 4. Health. I. Title: Dr. Gary Small's 14-day plan to keep your brain and body young. II. Vorgan, Gigi. III. Title.

QP406.S615 2004
153.1'2—dc22

2004040505

Hyperion books are available for special promotions and premiums. For details contact Michael Rentas, Manager, Inventory and Premium Sales, Hyperion, 77 West 66th Street, 11th floor, New York, New York 10023-6298, or call 212-456-0133.

FIRST EDITION

10 9 8 7 6 5 4 3 2 1

Acknowledgments

The Memory Prescription could not have been written without the love and support of our family, especially our children, Rachel and Harry, and our parents, Gertrude and Dr. Max Small, and Rose Vorgan-Weiss and Fred Weiss. We also appreciate the encouragement and insightful contributions we received from our extended family, friends, and colleagues, including Helen Berman, Karen Brocato, Rachel Champeau, Teresann Crowe-Lear, David DeNinno, Debbie Dorsey, Dr. Linda Ercoli, Dr. Howard Fillit, Mindy and Dr. Rob Gandin, Dr. David Heber, James Jennings, Andrea Kaplan, Jeffrey Nemerovski, Dr. Michael Phelps, Dr. John Schwartz, Dottie Sefton, Pauline Spaulding, Susan and Leon Tuberman, Roseanne and Maurice Wainer, and Mark Wilson. We were fortunate to have the assistance of renowned photographer Rena Small, and the help of several friends who displayed their hidden talent for modeling, including Cynthia Bougoukalos, Amy Gandin, Sheila and Andy Garb, Valerie and Stuart Grant, Dr. Shirley Impellizzeri, and Dr. Tom Marinaro. Once again, we were delighted to work with our gifted editor, Mary Ellen O'Neill, who helped us shape this book from the ground up, as well as Beth Dickey and the rest of our superb team at

Hyperion. Finally, we are deeply indebted to our dear friend and literary agent, Sandra Dijkstra, whose energy, guidance, and relentless support made *The Memory Prescription* a reality.

Gary Small
Gigi Vorgan

Contents

Preface   ix

Chapter One
Welcome to My Office   1

Chapter Two
Rate Your Current Mental and
Physical Fitness Level   16

Chapter Three
The 14-Day Memory Prescription   33

Chapter Four
Your 2-Week Checkup—
Gauge Your Success   103

Chapter Five
Pump Up Your Mental Aerobics   113

Contents

Chapter Six
Advanced Memory Training   139

Chapter Seven
Memory Prescription Diet—Eating for Longevity   161

Chapter Eight
Focus on Stress Reduction   190

Chapter Nine
Physical Fitness Jump-Start   214

Chapter Ten
Drugs and Supplements—Myths, Truths,
and Consequences   247

Chapter Eleven
Renewing Your Prescription—
A Lifetime of Quality Longevity   269

Appendixes
  1. *Suggested Grocery List for the Memory Prescription Diet*   287
  2. *Optional Recipes for the Memory Prescription Diet*   290
  3. *Sample Worksheets for Daily Progress Reports*   296
  4. *What to Do If Alzheimer's Disease Strikes*   298
  5. *Research Update and What's on the Horizon*   315
  6. *Glossary*   324
  7. *Additional Resources*   337

Bibliography   347
Permissions and Source Credits   355
Index   357

Preface

Many of today's health and conditioning programs emphasize physical strength and body image, but ignore the vital importance of brain fitness and mental acuity—which direct all our efforts to remain youthful, mentally fit, and at the top of our game. Of course, maintaining low cholesterol, watching our weight, and preventing high blood pressure all help to increase life expectancy. But research has shown that it first takes a healthy and agile brain to motivate us to treat our bodies right and achieve our highest quality longevity throughout each new phase of life.

In *The Memory Bible*, I introduced my recent discoveries and techniques for improving memory and keeping our brains young. Several readers commented that not only did the book's exercises and strategies improve their memory abilities, it made them feel younger—both mentally and physically. I was particularly struck by how many people who had committed to my four-pronged approach of stress reduction, healthy brain diet, memory exercises, and physical conditioning reported almost *immediate* results.

At the same time, I have received letters, phone calls, and e-mail requesting an even more detailed, customized, and simple "quick-start" plan—in a sense, a doctor's prescription—to propel individuals toward a sharper mind, more youthful body, and overall quality longevity—ASAP.

The Memory Prescription will give you just that—an aggressive, step-by-step program that brings immediate results and long-term benefits. Readers will feel as if they have entered my office to get their own private consultation and personally designed program, with our UCLA studies to back it up.

The 14-Day Memory Prescription allows you to experience not only improved mental and physical fitness, but also increased vitality and reduced levels of stress. If you stick with the Prescription, you'll notice enhanced recall abilities, feel younger and stronger, and look better overall. But wait, there's more! For no extra charge, I'll throw in a decrease in your odds of developing arthritis, heart disease, Alzheimer's disease, diabetes, and several other illnesses associated with aging.

If it's true that we are only as young as we feel, then every one of us can be younger in just 14 days.

Gary Small, M.D.
Los Angeles, California
May 2004

The Memory Prescription

Chapter One:

Welcome to My Office

If you want things to stay as they are, things will have to change.
—GIUSEPPE DI LAMPEDUSA

You're at a party with your wife when you spot a familiar face across the room. He waves. You know the guy but you can't recall his name. He starts toward you as you run the alphabet through your head—you're up to "L" and still no name comes to mind. He's two yards away with a giant grin on his face—M, N, O, P . . . He pumps your hand and says, "Gary! How the heck are you? You look great, Gary. Must be that clean living and Gigi's good cooking, huh? Nice to see you again too, Gigi." Gigi, equally stumped, stammers, "Nice to see *YOU*." You're sweating. He's already said your name three more times and *you* know that *he* knows that you've forgotten his. Just then your friend Sue walks up and you're saved! Surely she'll get his name. "Sue!" you bellow as if she were the last sip of water in the Sahara. You turn to the guy, "Have you met Sue?" He smiles and shakes her hand, "Haven't had the pleasure." Sue mumbles something about spicy stuffed mushrooms and walks off. The guy won't give you a break, and you've gone too far to ask his name now. Embarrassing? You bet. Uncommon? Not in the least.

Although memory challenges affect people of all ages, most of us complain of increasing forgetfulness as we age. To date, no one has yet located an actual "fountain of youth" on this planet, but I am among the billions awaiting a first sighting. In the meantime, I have spent several years developing a scientifically sound program to help my patients keep their brains and bodies young, and I present that program to you in this book.

Of course no one can escape getting older, but we can slow down the process and avoid many age-related conditions that may interfere with life's pleasures. My *14-Day Memory Prescription* (Chapter 3) will keep you on track by helping you focus on the four major areas where we can and must take control of our lives in order to achieve the highest quality longevity. The 14-Day Memory Prescription combines memory training, stress reduction, physical conditioning, and a healthy diet allowing you to dramatically improve your memory, health, and vitality. You will look and feel younger and sharper in just two weeks time.

It would be impossible to literally see every reader in my office to personally design their program; however, this book is organized to provide you with a similar experience. The 14-Day Memory Prescription lets you instantly begin your program for achieving *quality longevity*, which I define as remaining healthy, mentally fit, and youthful looking throughout a long and productive life.

Many of my patients are stressed-out high-achievers with multiple responsibilities at home and on the job. They often consult me because they have heard about research breakthroughs on healthy aging or new memory techniques, and they want to keep their brains and bodies in peak performance. Some contact me because they have already begun to experience mild memory changes or concerns; or perhaps they have relatives with Alzheimer's disease, prompting them to begin protecting their brains as early as possible.

People are sometimes mystified by how aging sneaks up on them. I often suggest imagining a slow-growing weed with four wily tendrils—stress, physical laziness, mental inactivity, and a bad fatty diet—growing in your garden. Left untended, these nasty tendrils begin wrapping around your healthy plants, strangling the youth and vitality right out of your flowers. Unless you become a responsible gardener, the aging weed can take over. Take the case of Michael C. . . .

Michael C. checks his watch—only 3:15 P.M. He rubs his tired eyes and pushes back from his desk. It's piled so high with briefs and depositions, he can hardly see the phone, which miraculously hasn't rung in over 30 seconds. He massages his neck, which feels like a rock from all the tension he's holding there—it kept him up half the night again. Glancing out the window, he sees two joggers turn the corner, and tries to remember where he put the number of that trainer Dr. Frank recommended. But hell, who's got time to work out anyway? Every lawyer on the eighth floor is vying for the partner promotion, and at 44, Michael's not the youngest rooster in the henhouse.

He crosses the hall to get some coffee and manages to snag the last glazed doughnut. It won't help lower his cholesterol, but he really needs some energy to get through the afternoon. Turning back to his office, Michael practically mows over Harrison J., Senior Partner and *Boss*, spilling coffee on his shoe. Michael apologizes but the Boss snaps, "Why weren't you at this morning's staff meeting?" Michael looks confused. "Isn't that tomorrow morning?" Boss laughs—and not very nicely. "Better have your memory checked, pal. You're developing a serious problem there. Hey, Jimmy-boy!" Boss calls to another associate and heads down the hall. Michael watches in pain—the slight migraine he's been staving off all day suddenly sets in, full force.

He didn't need a blunder like this—not now. And he *has* been forgetting a lot. His heart races as he heads for the safety of his office. The phone is ringing and three lines are flashing and as Michael tries not to hyperventilate, he remembers Dr. Frank saying, "Your cholesterol is sky-high. And you're under too much stress! Keep doing what you're doing and you'll be dead before you're 45!"

When Michael C. walked into my office soon after this experience, he was terrified about losing his ability to work and live normally. He said he couldn't concentrate and that he was losing his memory, and he was only 44. He wanted a full battery of psychological and neurological testing, and he desperately wanted to make sure he didn't have a brain tumor or some rare disease.

I asked Michael about his lifestyle—his dietary habits, physical conditioning, stress levels, workload, as well as his health history. He took a memory assessment test, and I checked for previous depression or anxiety problems. We discussed his health concerns including cholesterol and blood pressure control, and I did standard blood tests to make sure there were no immediate physical problems.

By the end of the assessment, it became clear that Michael C. was experiencing severe chronic stress. This stress was affecting his memory, as well as threatening his overall physical health. He needed a prescription, and I knew just what to write.

Michael C. left my clinic optimistic and self-assured. Although he didn't get the battery of unnecessary tests that he originally thought he needed, Michael left with something better—a personalized Memory Prescription that allowed him to immediately reduce his stress levels, improve his overall physical health, regain and improve his memory abilities, and begin a healthy longevity program to keep his brain and body young.

The latest scientific studies show that for all of us to achieve the highest level of quality longevity, we need to focus on the Big 4—the four most important areas to address if we are ever to slow, stop, or possibly reverse the aging process: mental activity, physical activity, stress reduction, and healthy eating. And, you get more bang for your buck—the results are better, faster, and longer lasting—when your efforts in these four areas are combined, as in the 14-Day Memory Prescription. The 14-Day Plan is an easy to follow, daily guide on what to eat, how to exercise mentally and physically, and how to minimize the chronic stress most of us live with today.

Just as I did for Michael C. in my office, this book will help you assess your own memory abilities, stress levels, physical conditioning, and dietary needs (Chapter 2). The 14-Day Memory Prescription is set up to begin on a Monday. The weekday menus and exercises vary from those of the weekends and progress throughout the course of the plan. The Prescription builds gradually over the 14 days, so it is easy to learn and integrate into your daily schedule. Although the 14-Day Memory Prescription is designed to meet the needs of nearly everyone, subsequent chapters will show you how to contour your program to best reach your specific healthy longevity goals.

But wait! You may be saying, "I don't want to read the whole book first! I want to start my 14 days to feeling and looking younger right now!" Then by all means, jump to page 33 and begin the 14-Day Memory Prescription today. This book works for all types of readers. Some readers may finish reading this book before starting their 14-Day Memory Prescription; others may want to jump right into Day One of the program as soon as they get the book home. *The Memory Prescription* is designed for everybody. Whatever your style may be at the beginning, the important thing is to begin.

Whether you are a working mother juggling a career, household, and carpool duties, a retired professional concerned with aging issues and increased forgetfulness, or perhaps a college student with upcoming finals and two part-time jobs, we all have stress in our lives, as well as room to improve our diets, physical conditioning, and general lifestyle choices. And we can all benefit from protecting our bodies and brains from the effects of aging. Those with legitimate concerns about inheriting an aging-related condition should know that genetic risk is not a guarantee that they will develop the condition. In fact, the sooner those people begin following their *Memory Prescription*—protecting their brain and body from the effects of aging—the more likely it is the conditions will *not* develop.

I've been asked why I created a 14-day plan, and not a 21-, or even a 28-day program. I have three reasons: First, the 14-Day Memory Prescription works—people see positive and significant results in 14 days or less. Second, two weeks is an undaunting commitment for most of us to make to a new program—even on a lark—such as picking up a catchy title we spot at the bookstore or perhaps notice somebody reading at a coffee bar. Third, I have found that when people continue my program for at least 14 days, they reach a critical milestone where they notice a real change occurring in their lives. They have given themselves just enough time to develop new brain and body fitness habits, which provide them momentum to stick with the plan for the long haul. And our UCLA research team has found that real, measurable changes in brain efficiency and true objective improvement in memory and mood occur in just 14 days.

An Ounce of Prevention

It's fairly easy to step on the scale or glance in the mirror to notice it's time to take off a few pounds or re-up your membership at the gym. And the doctor can be an effective motivator to change your diet by cutting out sugars, fats, or salt when he reports a ridiculously high cholesterol level or blood pressure reading. However, the signals are more subtle, less "in your face" if you will, that tell us it's time to jump-start our memory fitness programs and begin protecting our brains from the effects of aging.

Public education campaigns during the past few decades have led to declines in heart disease and stroke, and prevention efforts and improvements in early detection, treatment, and care have resulted in a number of beneficial trends, including a decline in cigarette smoking and a decrease in mean blood pressure levels in the U.S. population. Data from the National Health and Nutrition Examination Surveys suggest that decreases in the percentage of calories from dietary fat and the levels of dietary cholesterol correspond to decreases in blood cholesterol levels. Currently, the most frequently prescribed medicines throughout the world are those that lower blood cholesterol.

But the aging brain, that silent, hidden, ever-shrinking bundle of neurons and supporting tissue, with its insidious little clumps of plaque and tangles building up every day, is given the cold shoulder of denial by most people until it gets in our face and screams, "I'M IN TROUBLE!" And often, by then, it has already experienced irreparable damage, resulting in brain cell death.

A visit to the dermatologist for an injection or two may help iron out a few forehead wrinkles temporarily, but avoiding sun exposure and using sunscreen to impede skin aging in the first place is a better strategy. A surgeon may be able to cut out a cancer and prolong your life, but not smoking cigarettes is a more effective approach to living cancer-free. Despite rapidly advancing medical discoveries, in our lifetime, it will always be easier to protect your brain cells while they are healthy than to bring dead neurons back to life.

The Memory Fitness Movement

Current research findings and medical technological advances clearly support the principle of protecting both our bodies *and* our brains, yet there still exists no major brain-health awareness campaign or anti-Alzheimer's disease, public-health prevention program. Although many people joke about their memory slips, assigning them nicknames like "senior moments" or "middle-age pauses," sometimes the humor serves to mask an underlying fear and denial of the dreaded mental decline we have all witnessed in many older people. Too many still believe that it can't happen to them, at least not until they get much, much older.

But a revolution is afoot. A growing number of adults of all ages are realizing that we cannot keep our heads in the sand and assume that "they" will find a cure long before *we* lose our own memory and thinking abilities. People with little or no memory complaints are simply looking to perform and feel better, and remain at the top of their game. They want to take charge and remain healthy and mentally agile, and to prevent the illnesses their parents and grandparents suffered. These people are among the millions joining an international memory fitness movement in response to the growing scientific evidence that prevention may work as well for the brain as it has for the heart. Medical science is striving to keep us alive for 120 years, but what's the point if we can't enjoy that longevity with a mentally fit brain? The good news is, it's easier than one imagines to begin a memory fitness routine, and using a program like *The Memory Prescription* to protect your brain, benefits your body too.

Protecting Your Brain—
Never Too Late or Too Early

Most people combine busy lives with hectic schedules and multi-tasking—working, studying, caring for children or aging parents or both, managing finances, health-care, social engagements, and trying to fit in that daily workout. There is a whole lot to remember and plenty of opportunities to forget. It doesn't matter what age we are, we all face daily challenges of keeping our brains fit.

The scientific evidence is clear: brain aging begins as early as our twenties. Therefore it is never too early, and probably never too late, to fight off brain aging. Data show that as our neurons age and die, the actual overall size of the brain shrinks or atrophies. Also, aging brains accumulate lesions known as *amyloid plaques* and *neurofibrillary tangles*. This decayed material, resulting from cell death and degeneration of brain tissue, collects mainly in areas involved in memory and is believed to be responsible for Alzheimer's disease.

Neuropathological studies of plaques and tangles show that this physical evidence of brain decay begins to build up in the brain very early in adult life, for some people perhaps in their twenties and thirties. Our research at UCLA using the brain scanning technique known as positron emission tomography, or PET scanning, has uncovered Alzheimer's-like brain activity patterns in middle-aged people with hardly any memory complaints. As we follow these individuals with repeated PET scans, we find that their brain aging continues to advance over the years and the rate that it progresses is greater for people who have inherited a genetic risk for the disease from one of their parents.

The search to uncover what determines the rate at which our brains age and our risk for dementia has revealed a startling fact: for the average person, only about one-third of this determination comes from genetics. So if two thirds of what determines our future risk has to do with our environment and the lifestyle choices we make today, we clearly have more control over our future than many might imagine—two-thirds control.

To help diagnose subtle brain aging, we at UCLA have developed a *brain stress test* that works much like a cardiac stress test. Rather than walking uphill on a treadmill to stress the heart so the cardiogram can pick up any mild signs of heart disease, our functional magnetic resonance imaging (MRI) scanner detects subtle evidence of brain aging while volunteers stress their brains with memory tasks. Dr. Susan Bookheimer and I found that in middle-aged people with normal memory function but also the apolipoprotein E-4 (APOE-4) Alzheimer's risk gene, the brain had to work harder to perform a memory task than in people without a genetic risk. And the harder the brain worked during the initial test, the worse their memory function was two years later at the follow-up testing. The best explanation for these findings is that our brains naturally try to compensate for subtle deficits, but after a while, compensating no longer works and memory function worsens. However, brain-imaging studies show that this need not be our fate if we choose to do something about it.

Just by reading this book, you are already doing something to change this unnecessary scenario. Hopefully you are like many of my patients, some of whom may be noticing very subtle memory changes, who want to fight back and take control by conditioning and training their brains. Some refer to themselves as the "worried well."

Dr. Richard Heir and associates at the University of California, Irvine, performed PET scans while young volunteers in their twenties played a then novel computer game called Tetris. At first, their brain scans showed lots of brain activity, indicating that they used up a lot of brain energy despite dismal scores on the game. After a month or so of practice, the volunteers became Tetris experts, while their brain scans showed minimal if any activity during play. In just weeks, they had developed significant brain efficiency, allowing for increased memory capacity and greater ease in solving memory problems.

Dr. Heir's research suggests that even as early as our twenties we can become proactive and increase our brain efficiency. More recent studies also argue for an early start to memory fitness strategies. Dr. Daniel Silverman and I looked at the PET scans of young adults with normal memory abilities and compared their brain function according to whether or not they finished college plus the added effect of whether they did or did not have the Alzheimer's APOE-4 genetic risk. We found that during mental rest, the scans revealed the greatest brain activity in the group that had *completed* college and did *not* have the APOE-4 gene. Those young adults who did *not* complete college and did *not* have the APOE-4 gene, or who had completed college and *did* carry the APOE-4 gene, showed an intermediate level of brain activity. We found the least amount of brain activity during mental rest in the group that did *not* complete college and *did* carry the APOE-4 gene.

It is interesting that the influence of a college education on a person's brain activity reserve was even more powerful than that of the APOE-4 risk gene. Ideally, someone concerned about their genetic risk could compensate for possible brain activity deficits through further education.

So getting started early makes sense. When would be too late? Unless someone is already suffering from late-stage dementia or severe Alzheimer's disease, a program of mental activity, physical conditioning, stress reduction, and healthy diet will likely improve an individual's daily functioning, overall health, and quality of life. Of course, these kinds of strategies will have less impact on patients with progressed conditions.

Dr. Fred Gage of the Salk Institute in La Jolla, California, has found that new nerve growth, or neurogenesis, is possible in adult human brains. I know of several senior scientists who are now working to develop intensive mental stimulation interventions designed to arouse brain cell function and improve cognitive abilities. They believe that the basic laboratory studies show that the "use it or lose it" theory may hold true even for patients who have already developed dementia. Many of us agree that it is never too late to jump-start an individual's brain fitness.

Everyone should begin and maintain a memory fitness program without delay, especially in light of new, alarming research on the projected prevalence of Alzheimer's disease. Currently, about 4.5 million people have Alzheimer's in the United States. Researchers at Rush-Presbyterian-St. Luke's Medical Center in Chicago recently reported that by the year 2050, over 13 million older Americans will suffer from Alzheimer's disease unless we find new ways to prevent or treat it.

I am among the many scientists optimistic that we can change the course of this epidemic. We now have the technologies to make significant advances in the next five to ten years in the development of more effective treatments, particularly preventive interventions. But even before these advances take effect, we already have a considerable arsenal to stave off brain aging and decelerate memory decline as we age. Mounting scientific evidence is pointing the way for us to change our lifestyles to protect our brains.

Boot Camp for the Brain

When I think of a boot camp, I imagine a training environment where the goal is accelerated learning of new strategies, tactics, and routines. The camp provides all the instruction and structure needed to allow "campers" to simply do as they're told and soak up the benefits of the training. The 14-Day Memory Prescription is like boot camp "lite"—it's easy to do but has a great impact, lasting only two weeks and resulting in significant benefits that can sustain themselves well beyond that time. It pulls together the Big 4 proven strategies for brain and body health—mental activity, physical conditioning, stress reduction, and the healthy brain diet—and delivers them in a simple yet intensive "boot camp for the brain."

At UCLA, we have been documenting the benefits of this kind of focused intervention using the latest brain imaging technologies; however, we observed the plan's positive results even without the high tech devices. Our volunteers were effusive about how much better they felt. Their memory test scores and personal testimonials were convincing, and we could see it in their facial expressions and the way they carried themselves.

Sandra B., a 41-year-old legal assistant, suffered from chronic low-back pain over the years and had tried lots of traditional and non-traditional remedies without much success. She began the 14-Day Memory Prescription program skeptical that two weeks of altering her diet and exercise routines could really do much for her. She was only mildly aware of any memory issues, but wrote them off to being distracted by her back pain. A quiet and reserved person, Sandra never seemed too enthusiastic about things, nor did she complain much. When asked to rate herself on a scale from 1 to 10—1 the worst and 10 the best—on how she felt overall before starting the plan, she thought for a moment and said, "6."

After completing the program, Sandra rated herself a 9. She looked brighter and more alert, and said she had lost three pounds. She had begun bicycle riding after work with her neighbor and the stretching component of the plan had even helped her back.

Bill G. was eager to give the program a try. He was stressed out at work, had difficulty remembering details, and his doctor was concerned about his cholesterol and blood pressure. Bill had dabbled in yoga classes before, had joined a fitness center, and done Weight Watchers, but he always had trouble staying on his various wellness programs. He said he was so busy at his office he didn't want to take on a fitness program where he had to do any work or feel like he was taking on another "job." What appealed to him about the 14-Day Memory Prescription was that everything was laid out in detail. Nothing was left to chance—no big decisions or choices to make unless he wanted to. The Memory Prescription told him what to eat and drink, when to stretch, what memory fitness exercises to do, and when to relax.

After the initial two-week program, Bill's subjective and objective memory scores improved, and he stopped complaining about misplacing his keys and glasses. To his surprise, he was able to lose five pounds and keep it off, even though the program had him eating breakfast every day for a change. He and his wife looked forward to their brisk walk after dinner each evening, and he had even lowered his cholesterol. Bill asked me if I could give him a six-month program and I suggested he simply renew his Memory Prescription. The lifestyle changes he made in those first two weeks can and should become healthy life-long habits.

The Memory Prescription Study

We had many people like Sandra and Bill volunteer for our UCLA study, to help us prove to ourselves, and the scientific community, that the Memory Prescription works. In this controlled research program, we recruit people with mild memory complaints, ranging in age from 35 to 80. Before they begin, we check their memory scores, mood, physical health, and many other measures. We gauge their level of stress and whether they are overweight. In fact, we have them complete the same assessments that you will complete in Chapter 2.

In the study, we also perform more detailed memory tests, measure blood pressure and cholesterol levels, and determine the volunteers' level of brain efficiency using the functional MRI brain stress test and the PET scan. After two weeks on the program we repeat all these assessments. To control for the possible "placebo effect" from all these assessment procedures and brain scans, we have a second group of volunteers undergo the same assessments but simply continue their ordinary lifestyle habits for the 14 days. To prove that the program works, we compare the two groups on their baseline, as well as their two-week test scores and scan results.

In our initial assessment of results, after just two weeks of Memory Prescription, volunteers demonstrated improved memory performance and brain efficiency. During the brain stress test, not only did they score better on the memory tasks, but they also used less brainpower to do it—just as an athlete eventually exerts less energy but lifts heavier weights or runs farther after continued physical training.

Each individual element of the program, from physical conditioning to stress reduction, can improve your brain and body fitness. But putting them all together, as the Memory Prescription does, creates a synergy that goes well beyond their individual impact. In other words, the sum is greater than the parts.

Scientists have observed this kind of synergy in other studies. For example, investigators at the National Public Health Institute in Finland studied how a healthy diet combined with physical exercise affects the risk for diabetes. They found that losing as few as 10 pounds and eating a healthy diet, while exercising regularly, reduced the risk for developing type-2 diabetes by more than 50 percent.

Duke University researchers looked at how cardiac patients were affected by combining stress reduction strategies with a physical activity program. The study found that the group who exercised *and* learned anger management techniques ended up with the lowest risk for ischemic chest pain, which results from insufficient blood flow and oxygen to the heart. The group of patients who merely exercised and did *not* have anger management instruction lowered their risk for chest pain slightly, but only half as much as the other group. The physiological process leading to this kind of diminished blood flow in the heart has the potential for producing similar circulatory problems in the brain.

By employing the Memory Prescription's synergistic approach, you will not only begin to feel better, more confident, and younger, but you will have begun to literally change how your brain functions, making it more efficient and improving your memory.

Refill Your Prescription for Life

Although the initial 14 days of the Memory Prescription is enough time to "jump-start" your brain and body into new healthy habits, most people are so pleased with their initial results that they decide to stick with the program for months and years to come.

After completing the 14-Day Plan, you will possess the tools, motivation, and know-how to continue your newly developed quality longevity habits into the future. If you wish to make adjustments to one or more of the elements of your program—stress reduction, mental conditioning, healthy brain diet, or physical fitness—subsequent chapters throughout the book will guide you on how best to personalize your Prescription to get the most benefits from it. The Appendixes will provide more detail on recipe options and other informative resources.

Although *The Memory Prescription* is not a sequel to my last book, *The Memory Bible*, it does take its healthy brain and body objectives to the next level by laying out exactly how to achieve them. *The Memory Prescription* will allow you to skip that trek to my office and launch your healthy longevity program today.

Chapter Two:

Rate Your Current Mental and Physical Fitness Level

*If you want to test your memory, try to recall
what you were worrying about one year ago today.*
— ROTARIAN

As we do in my clinic, this chapter will help you rate your current memory fitness levels. We will assess your objective and subjective memory abilities and your daily stress levels, and we will determine your baseline physical stamina status. Your scores on these assessments will allow you to gauge your improvements after just two weeks on the plan, when you will be given a second opportunity to assess your levels and compare those with your baseline scores.

Evaluating your current mental and physical fitness levels also can be pivotal in tailoring the basic 14-Day Memory Prescription to meet any specific needs you may have. By the end of this chapter, you'll know whether your program should include extra stress reduction techniques, more advanced memory training, or maybe additional aerobic conditioning, or alterations to your healthy brain diet such as additional weight loss strategies.

The assessment tests after the initial two-week program are equally valuable. Our UCLA study subjects showed definite improvements in memory performance and mood levels after completing the 14-Day Memory Prescription, and they scored higher on follow-up assessments on nearly all the areas we measured. Researchers have shown that such self-awareness of personal improvement is very empowering. It gives us confidence in our memory skills, and that added sense of confidence helps us perform even better over time.

Assessing Memory Ability

When designing a memory fitness plan, it is important to assess memory both objectively (how well you actually perform on a memory test) and subjectively (how good you perceive your own memory abilities to be).

Objective memory ratings from pencil and paper tests tell us important information about brain fitness and health. For example, in our UCLA research we found that people having verbal difficulties (retrieving words, remembering names, etc.) often show decreased brain function activity on PET (positron emission tomography) scans, mainly in the left hemisphere, which is the side of the brain known to control language and verbal abilities. Similarly, people with visual and spatial memory difficulties (recalling directions, gauging distances, etc.) generally show deficits in the right hemisphere, the side of the brain that controls visual and spatial functions.

Higher objective memory scores (pencil and paper tests) tend to predict continued good results on future tests, and minimal, if any, decline in brain function over time. Few of us realize, however, that subjective reports of memory change, or how we feel about our own memory abilities, are also significant predictors of whether or not our memory function will or will not decline over time. Studies indicate that middle-aged and older people whose subjective memory loss is minimal or nil, do in fact score higher on objective memory tests than those reporting greater self-awareness of memory loss.

Some degree of self-awareness of memory change is expected as we age. And it's often a good thing, especially if it motivates us to do something about it, such as starting the 14-Day Memory Prescription. According to our studies, the 14-Day Plan can lead to significant improvements in both objective and subjective memory performance in as little as two weeks. And by integrating the Memory Prescription into your daily lifestyle, you will not only be protecting your brain and body from the effects of aging, you will be doing all you can to guarantee yourself the highest quality longevity possible. You don't have to take my word for it—your future assessment scores will prove it.

Rate Your Subjective Memory Ability

The best way to learn how aware you are of your own memory changes is to answer a series of straightforward questions, and neuropsychologists have developed standardized questionnaires for just this purpose. On the following pages, you will find a shortened version of the assessment tool developed by Dr. Michael Gilewski and his associates at Cedars-Sinai Medical Center in Los Angeles. My research group has used this rating system extensively and found it reflects true memory changes as well as other subtle aspects of brain function.

Take out a pencil and answer the following questions by circling a number between 1 and 7 that best reflects how you judge your own memory ability. By tallying the results of your completed questionnaire, you will then have a baseline of your current memory self-ratings—your "before" scores—taken just prior to beginning the 14-Day Plan. After two weeks on the plan, you will be given an opportunity to repeat the test, compare results, and gauge your improvement for yourself.

SUBJECTIVE MEMORY QUESTIONNAIRE

	Poor	Good	Excellent
How would you rate your overall memory?	1 2	3 4 5	6 7

	Always	Sometimes	Never
How often do these present a problem for you?			
names	1 2	3 4 5	6 7
faces	1 2	3 4 5	6 7
appointments	1 2	3 4 5	6 7

where I put things (e.g., keys, eyeglasses)	1	2	3	4	5	6	7
performing household chores	1	2	3	4	5	6	7
directions to places	1	2	3	4	5	6	7
phone numbers I have just checked	1	2	3	4	5	6	7
phone numbers I use frequently	1	2	3	4	5	6	7
things people tell me	1	2	3	4	5	6	7
keeping up correspondence	1	2	3	4	5	6	7
personal dates (e.g., birthdays)	1	2	3	4	5	6	7
words	1	2	3	4	5	6	7
forgetting what I wanted to buy at the store	1	2	3	4	5	6	7
taking a test	1	2	3	4	5	6	7
beginning something and forgetting what I was doing	1	2	3	4	5	6	7
losing my thread of thought in conversation	1	2	3	4	5	6	7
losing my thread of thought in public speaking	1	2	3	4	5	6	7
knowing whether I have already told someone something	1	2	3	4	5	6	7

As you read a novel, how often do you have trouble remembering what you have read . . .	Always		Sometimes			Never	
in opening chapters, once I've finished the book?	1	2	3	4	5	6	7
3 or 4 chapters before the one I'm now reading?	1	2	3	4	5	6	7
in the chapter before the one I'm now reading?	1	2	3	4	5	6	7
in the paragraph just before the one I'm now reading?	1	2	3	4	5	6	7

	Poorly		Fair		Well	

in the sentence just before the one
   I'm now reading?   **1 2   3 4 5   6 7**

How well do you remember things which occurred ...   **Poorly   Fair   Well**

last month?   **1 2   3 4 5   6 7**

between six months and one year ago?   **1 2   3 4 5   6 7**

between one and five years ago?   **1 2   3 4 5   6 7**

between six and ten years ago?   **1 2   3 4 5   6 7**

When you read a newspaper or magazine
article, how often do you have trouble
remembering what you have read ...   **Always   Sometimes   Never**

in the opening paragraphs, once I have
   finished the article?   **1 2   3 4 5   6 7**

3 or 4 paragraphs before the one I am
   currently reading?   **1 2   3 4 5   6 7**

in the paragraph before the one I am
   currently reading?   **1 2   3 4 5   6 7**

3 or 4 sentences before the one I am
   currently reading?   **1 2   3 4 5   6 7**

in the sentence before the one I am
   currently reading?   **1 2   3 4 5   6 7**

Subjective Memory Total Score, Baseline: _____

Add up all the numbers you have circled and write in your sum above. A total score of 200 or higher indicates your subjective memory difficulties are minimal. If you master the memory training exercises in the basic 14-Day Plan fairly quickly, you may wish to introduce more advanced memory exercises into your program (Chapter 6).

A total score between 100 and 200 suggests that you are noticing a slight to moderate degree of memory change. The memory training exercises included in the basic 14-Day Memory Prescription vary in degree of difficulty and some people in this score range may require extra time to complete the more demanding exercises. It is also possible to modify them so they are less challenging in the beginning (Chapter 6). For example, if a particular memory exercise lists six words to remember at a session, you might want to work only on the first four words.

A total score below 100 reflects an even greater self-awareness of memory difficulties and implies that memory training will be a larger challenge. It will be important to take your time with each memory exercise and to stick with the program. You might consider contacting your physician about these concerns, or perhaps one of the experts in your area (Appendix 7).

Whatever your score on this first assessment, keep in mind this is simply your baseline—once you have completed two weeks on the Memory Prescription, your score will go up.

Assess Your Objective Memory Ability

To get an even better idea of how well your memory is working, we'll need to do an objective memory quiz to assess your current learning and recall abilities. Because the traditional, extensive forms of objective memory assessments—neuropsychological testing—can take hours, sometimes even days, to complete and require highly trained professionals to administer, score, and interpret, I have developed a simple, do-it-yourself objective memory rating method that you can complete right now. This brief version of the more extensive assessment that we use in our work at UCLA emphasizes recall of words you will learn during the test. And recall—the ability to retrieve or pull information out of your memory storage—is *the* major area of concern for most people.

Don't be discouraged if you find this memory assessment method either too easy or too difficult. It is designed to assess memory in people with a wide range of abilities. I attempted to make it challenging enough so that most people will see concrete results from their memory skills training soon after getting started. You can expect your score to improve within the first week of your program.

Because the assessment is timed, you will need a stopwatch, kitchen timer, or timepiece with a second hand before beginning. The test involves learning a list of 10 words over a 2-minute period and recalling them after a 20-minute break. When ready, set your timer for two minutes, then read and learn the words on the list in Objective Memory Assessment No. 1.

OBJECTIVE MEMORY ASSESSMENT NO. 1
STUDY THE FOLLOWING WORDS
FOR UP TO TWO MINUTES:

Violin

Balloon

Stereo

Building

Strawberry

Cradle

Mast

Lizard

Teacher

Oven

When your two minutes are up, put aside *The Memory Prescription*, reset your timer for a 20-minute break, and do something else—return some phone calls, read the movie section of the newspaper, whatever you like, just make sure you distract yourself from the word list with something else. After the 20 minutes, write down as many of the words as you can recall and record the total number below:

Objective Memory Total Score, Baseline: _____

If you did well on your objective memory recall score (8 or greater), then the basic memory skills in the 14-Day Plan will probably be quite easy for you to master and you may want to add on some advanced memory skill training (Chapter 6). If your score is less than 8, then you will find that learning the basic memory skills in the 14-Day Plan will likely improve your performance. If your score is lower, below 4, you needn't panic—the program can be adjusted to slowly improve your scores.

This assessment tool is designed to be difficult for many people. You will get a chance to retest yourself after the 14-Day Plan, when most people will see obvious improvement. If your objective memory-recall score improves, then continue to build your memory skills program over time. If not, you might consider contacting your physician or an expert in your area for a professional evaluation (Appendix 7).

Age and level of educational achievement are among the many factors that can influence your objective memory score. In general, younger people score better than older people, and people who have had more educational experience will have better scores. Your scores are just an indicator or guide, not the last word, on your current brain fitness.

The pattern of your memory assessment scores can help us to individualize your Memory Prescription. Ironically, when we worry about memory performance our actual objective performance goes down. People familiar with Alzheimer's disease due to afflicted friends and relatives often fret over each of their own memory slips. This kind of excess worry about memory changes may actually worsen one's objective memory performance. If you scored well on the objective word recall after 20 minutes but your subjective memory score indicated frequent memory difficulties, you may be suffering from unnecessary stress and anxiety. I suggest augmenting the stress reduction component of your memory prescription (Chapter 8).

INTERPRETING SUBJECTIVE AND OBJECTIVE MEMORY SCORES—DETERMINING THE LEVEL TO BEGIN YOUR PROGRAM

| MEMORY SCORE | | Program |
Subjective	Objective	
High	High	Augment memory training with more advanced exercises as desired (Chapter 6).
High	Low	You may be unaware of some of your memory changes. Take time and focus on basic training. Reassess score and consult expert if no improvement.
Low	Low	Take time and focus on basic training, then reassess score. If no improvement, consult expert.
Low	High	Augment 14-Day Plan with additional stress reduction approaches (Chapter 8). Reassess score and consult expert if no improvement.

Are You Stressed Out?

You return from a much-needed week's vacation in the tropics—where you didn't take your laptop. You are relaxed, suntanned, and your wife's hero for making a hat out of palm fronds *and* ordering dinner in broken Tahitian. There is no way this serene and blissful feeling is going to wear off, even after going back to the grind at the office next week. You vow to rise above it, remember the tranquil waves of paradise, no matter how stressful the situation around you. And you do, until about noon your first day back at work.

The greatest hidden enemy of memory and quality longevity is chronic stress. High anxiety and stress levels often creep up on us without our awareness. Many of us lead tense and hurried lives, where even the mental and physical benefits of occasional rest and recreation disappear quickly and leave us as stressed out as before.

Everyone has a different baseline stress level, depending on personality style, coping skills, degree of self-awareness, and other factors. To get a better idea of how stressed out you are right now, complete the following stress level questionnaire, which I designed to assist in adjusting the 14-Day Plan for those requiring additional stress release exercises. Most people have found that their stress levels are gradually yet dramatically reduced as a result of the 14-Day Plan, and you will be able to assess this for yourself after two weeks.

STRESS LEVEL QUESTIONNAIRE

	Low		Medium			High	
How would you rate your overall stress level?	1	2	3	4	5	6	7

	Little		Somewhat			Very	
To what degree do the following situations make you tense or irritable?							
argument with friend or relative	1	2	3	4	5	6	7
waiting for a table in a restaurant	1	2	3	4	5	6	7
arriving late for an appointment	1	2	3	4	5	6	7
forgetting someone's name	1	2	3	4	5	6	7
anticipating work deadlines	1	2	3	4	5	6	7
last minute change in plans	1	2	3	4	5	6	7

	Easy		Medium			Difficult	
How easy is it for you to relax when you . . .							
watch a television show or movie?	1	2	3	4	5	6	7
read a book or magazine?	1	2	3	4	5	6	7
take a walk, jog, or do other physical exercise?	1	2	3	4	5	6	7

How often do you experience each of the following?	Never		Sometimes			Always	
insomnia	1	2	3	4	5	6	7
shortness of breath	1	2	3	4	5	6	7
rapid heart rate	1	2	3	4	5	6	7
cold hands or feet	1	2	3	4	5	6	7
impatience	1	2	3	4	5	6	7
irritability	1	2	3	4	5	6	7
indecisiveness	1	2	3	4	5	6	7
tension or worry	1	2	3	4	5	6	7

Add up your total score, which can range from 18 to 126, and record it below:

Stress Level Total Score, Baseline: _____

If your score is less than 40, then your stress levels are currently manageable; however, you will benefit from the stress release exercises in the basic 14-Day Plan. If you scored between 41 and 80, then you are experiencing the mid-range of stress levels. The 14-Day Plan will help you relax more readily throughout the day, which should allow you to be more focused when you are trying to learn new information or recall stored memories. If you scored between 81 and 126, then you are in the high-stress group and should review Chapter 8 to augment the stress reduction component of your plan. If you find that your stress levels do not diminish after the first two weeks, you might consider consulting with a physician about your challenges with chronic stress, how it may be affecting your health, and what else you can do about it.

Assess Your Level of Physical Fitness

Recent discoveries indicate that good physical conditioning protects and improves brain health and even lowers our eventual risk for developing Alzheimer's disease. Physical fitness and sports often figure into the lives of children and young adults. However, a majority of us fail to keep up daily exercise routines as job and family responsibilities squeeze out free time. The 14-Day Plan is designed to be safe and effective for people within a broad range of baseline physical activity levels, even those who have minimal or no physical fitness routine schedule in place.

Knowing your baseline fitness level will help you to tailor the aerobic conditioning component of your program to meet your specific needs now. Complete the following questionnaire by circling the number from 1 to 7, for each question, that best describes your current physical fitness level.

PHYSICAL FITNESS QUESTIONNAIRE

To what degree might the following activities make you feel short of breath?	Minimal		Somewhat		Very	
playing table tennis for 10 minutes	1 2		3 4 5		6 7	
walking briskly for 10 minutes	1 2		3 4 5		6 7	
jogging for 10 minutes	1 2		3 4 5		6 7	
climbing a flight of stairs	1 2		3 4 5		6 7	
climbing three flights of stairs	1 2		3 4 5		6 7	

How sore would you be after each of the following activities?	Minimal		Somewhat		Very	
sweeping floors for 10 minutes	1 2		3 4 5		6 7	
carrying grocery bags for 10 minutes	1 2		3 4 5		6 7	

carrying a 20-pound suitcase for 10 minutes	1	2	3	4	5	6	7
riding a bicycle for 30 minutes	1	2	3	4	5	6	7
playing two sets of tennis	1	2	3	4	5	6	7

Add up your total score, which can range from 10 to 70, and record it below:

Physical Fitness Total Score, Baseline: _____

A score below 25 suggests that you are in good physical condition. You can follow the 14-Day Memory Prescription plan without modification or you may wish to increase your physical activity levels by adding additional exercises (Chapter 9). If you scored in the moderate range (26 to 45), the 14-Day Plan should help you build up your stamina gradually while causing minimal soreness or overexertion. If you scored greater than 50, you might consider a discussion with your doctor before beginning the program. When starting the plan, you may want to build up your physical stamina more gradually than recommended in the basic plan by modifying it slightly, possibly by reducing the repetitions in each set of exercises (Chapter 9).

The Memory Prescription Diet

The Memory Prescription Diet for healthy brains and bodies, as presented in the 14-Day Plan, is designed for most people within an average range of body weights. However, several volunteers in our research studies lost weight while on the basic 14-Day Memory Prescription program. Some readers may wish assistance in shedding additional pounds. Modifications can be made to the Memory Prescription Diet to accommodate everyone's needs (Chapter 7). The charts below will help to determine if you are a candidate for modifications to the basic 14-Day Memory Prescription Diet.

The following tables indicate ideal weights according to height, sex, and body frame, adapted from data developed by the Metropolitan Life Insurance Company (1983). People with these particular body frames and heights, ages 25 to 59 years, were found to have the lowest mortality rates when their body weights were in these ideal ranges. If your weight is above the ideal range for your height and frame, you may want to adjust your Memory Prescription Diet as described in Chapter 7.

Use these tables as a guide, and check with your physician if you are unsure about whether or not you ought to lose weight.

IDEAL BODY WEIGHTS FOR WOMEN

Height	Small Frame	Medium Frame	Large Frame
4'9"	99–108	106–118	115–128
4'10"	100–110	108–120	117–131
4'11"	101–112	110–123	119–134
5'0"	103–115	112–126	122–137
5'1"	105–118	115–129	125–140
5'2"	108–121	118–132	128–144
5'3"	111–124	121–135	131–148
5'4"	114–127	124–138	134–152
5'5"	117–130	127–141	137–156
5'6"	120–133	130–144	140–160
5'7"	123–136	133–147	143–164
5'8"	126–139	136–150	146–167
5'9"	129–142	139–153	149–170
5'10"	132–145	142–156	152–173
5'11"	135–148	145–159	155–176

IDEAL BODY WEIGHTS FOR MEN

Height	Small Frame	Medium Frame	Large Frame
5'1"	123–129	126–136	133–145
5'2"	125–131	128–138	135–148
5'3"	127–133	130–140	137–151
5'4"	129–135	132–143	139–155
5'5"	131–137	134–161	141–159
5'6"	133–140	137–149	144–163
5'7"	135–143	140–152	147–167
5'8"	137–146	143–155	150–171
5'9"	139–149	146–158	153–175
5'10"	141–152	149–161	156–179
5'11"	144–155	152–165	159–183
6'0"	147–159	155–169	163–187
6'1"	150–163	159–173	167–192
6'2"	153–167	162–177	171–197
6'3"	157–171	166–182	176–202

Baseline Body Weight: _____

Even if your height and weight chart suggests you should drop a few pounds, I generally recommend that you first try the 14-Day Plan without any dietary adjustments. The aerobic exercise component combined with the Memory Prescription Diet's balance of healthy carbohydrates, fats, and proteins may be enough to initiate a modest weight reduction program. If you find that you haven't lost weight after the initial 14 days, then you may want to make some dietary adjustments as you renew your Memory Prescription for the next two weeks. Also, review Chapter 7 if you have any medical conditions such as diabetes, hypertension, or high cholesterol that may require special dietary needs.

Following Your Progress—
Charting Baselines for Setting Goals

After 14 days on the Memory Prescription plan, our UCLA research volunteers showed improvement in many, if not all, of the measures—particularly subjective and objective memory performance and stress and physical conditioning levels. An added benefit came when people became aware of their progress—their motivation to continue the program, or renew their Memory Prescription, increased greatly.

Now see for yourself. In the figure below, plot your initial, or baseline, scores for subjective and objective memory performance, stress and physical conditioning levels, and height/frame body weight range. After you complete the 14-Day Plan, you will have an opportunity to repeat these assessments and fill in the bottom line of this chart, thus comparing your scores. I'm confident you will see remarkable progress in each area of your life where you can take control and keep your brain and body young.

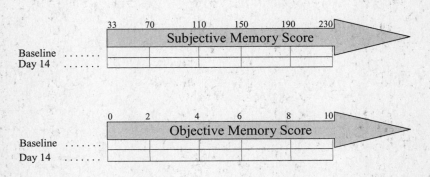

126	100	80	60	40	18
		Stress Level Score			

Baseline ....

Day 14 ....

70	55	47	35	22	10
		Physical Fitness Score			

Baseline ....

Day 14 ....

Body Weight	
Body Weight	*Height/Frame Body Weight Range*

Baseline ....

Day 14 ....

Chapter Three:

The 14-Day Memory Prescription

The reason I have such a good memory for names is because I took that Sam Carnegie course.
— ANTHONY QUINN

When I design a healthy longevity program, I try to keep it simple enough to begin immediately, yet flexible enough to stick with for a lifetime. Everybody's lifestyle should encompass a plan to keep their brain and body young, no matter what their age. These types of programs often first appeal to people who are beginning to experience mild memory complaints, perhaps a heightened level of daily stress, possibly a degree of physical fitness decline, or a combination of the above.

This chapter will show you how to manage the Big 4, the four most important areas in our lives to address in order to slow, stop, or possibly reverse the aging process: mental activity, healthy brain and body diet, stress reduction, and physical conditioning. Beginning with Day One, you will find specific daily recommendations on what to do, when to do it, and how—down to when to drink that next glass of water—in order to facilitate achieving your highest quality longevity goals. I have included clear and concise instructions with each new mental aerobics game, stretching and conditioning exercise, healthy brain and body diet tip, and stress reduction or "stress release" technique. As you become familiar with the basics, the plan will build on these skills.

A Few Tips Before Beginning

The 14-Day Memory Prescription is designed to meet the needs of most people. If desired, you will find ways to adjust the basic plan to fit most comfortably into your lifestyle. For example, if your schedule one day is too hectic to spare a few minutes for an afternoon mental aerobics exercise or stress release break, you could modify the program by performing them that evening at home, when you are less hurried.

The plan's healthy brain and body diet includes a nutritious balance of proteins and carbohydrates, as well as adequate quantities of foods rich in antioxidants and omega-3 fats. Recommended portions may be adjusted to suit your appetite needs. If you find that the portions are too small and you are experiencing undesired weight loss on the diet, simply increase your portions to remain at a stable body weight. If losing weight is one of your goals, see the *Losing Weight* section in Chapter 7 for guidance. Consider consulting your physician before embarking on this or any diet and exercise program.

Glance ahead at the next day or two's food selections for any shopping you may need to do. If you prefer to do your shopping for each week in advance, go to Appendix 1 for a weekly shopping list. I recommend marketing on Sunday prior to both the first and second Mondays of the 14-Day Memory Prescription Plan. Check to see what vitamin supplements you already have and which you will need to buy (Appendix 1) before beginning the program. Daily vitamins include 1 multi-vitamin, 500 mgs of vitamin C, 400 IUs of vitamin E, and 1,000 mgs of omega-3 fatty acid at breakfast. Some people like to augment their antioxidant vitamins in the evening by taking an additional 500 mgs of vitamin C and 400 IUs of vitamin E at dinner.

Optional food substitutions are described on page 101. Suggested optional recipes, marked by an asterisk (*) in the 14-Day Plan, are listed in Appendix 2. One or two alcoholic beverages in the evening are allowed on the plan.

The mental aerobics exercises included in the plan may be challenging for some and somewhat easier for others. If you find a particular exercise to be too frustrating, skip it and move on. With practice you will likely improve.

You may also want to refer to Chapter 5 to work on additional beginning level mental aerobic exercises.

You will learn my basic memory techniques, including LOOK, SNAP, CONNECT. If you'd like further explanation of this technique and more advanced memory methods, see Chapter 6.

The physical conditioning and stretching movements included in the plan are safe for most people and should be done at your own pace. If in doubt, consult your physician. Try to get a good night's sleep before embarking on the 14-Day Plan, and every night thereafter. Insomniacs, see Chapter 8 for tips on good sleep hygiene and its impact on memory performance.

The 14-Day Plan

1ST MONDAY (DAY ONE)

Tip for the Day: Our bodies and minds achieve peak performance when we are relaxed and stress-free. Purposely avoid one sure-fire stressful situation today. For example, leave five minutes early for work so a little unexpected traffic won't raise your blood pressure. Even if you don't notice the immediate benefits, stress reduction has a strong impact on long-term brain and body health.

WAKE-UP STRETCH AND CONDITIONING (1ST MONDAY)

Stretch #1 [*Deep Breathing Dips*] Stand with feet forward and shoulder width apart. Bend your knees slightly as you begin a deep breath, raising your arms out at your sides. Continue raising your arms, stretching them overhead until your fingertips touch, and your legs are straight. Exhale slowly while lowering your arms to your sides. Repeat 4 times.

Conditioning Exercise #1 [*Russian Dancer Knee Lifts*] Stand upright and fold your arms in front at shoulder height like a Russian folk dancer. Lift your right knee toward your right elbow, and then alternate your left knee toward your left elbow. Exhale as the knee comes up. Repeat for a count of 20.

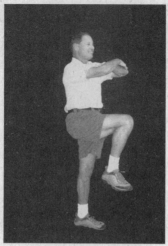

Russian Dancer Knee Lifts

Drink a glass of water.

BREAKFAST (1ST MONDAY)

Vegetable omelet (use 1 whole egg plus 2 egg whites)
½ cup fresh or frozen blueberries
Tea (green is best), coffee, water, or sparkling juice (1 part fruit juice plus 2
parts seltzer or soda water, over ice)
Vitamin supplements: 1 multivitamin; vitamin C—500 mgs; vitamin E—
400 IUs; omega-3 fatty acid—1,000 mgs

CAFFEINE ADDICTS *(you know who you are) refer to Caffeine Reduction
section in Chapter 7.*

MORNING MENTAL AEROBICS (1ST MONDAY)

Before leaving home, focus on two random details of the clothing or accessories on a family member, roommate, or the first person you see that day. Write those details on a piece of paper and slip it into your wallet.

FITNESS ON THE RUN (1ST MONDAY)

Park or get dropped off at a distance from your first destination of the day and walk briskly the rest of the way.

OR: If time allows, take a **5-minute** (or longer) morning walk.

Drink a glass of water.

MID-MORNING SNACK (1ST MONDAY)

½ cup nonfat plain or flavored yogurt with 1 tablespoon raisins
Green tea or water

MID-MORNING MENTAL AEROBICS (1ST MONDAY)

Write your first name using your left hand if you are right-handed, or vice-versa. Now, using *two* pencils, write your first name using both hands at the same time.

LUNCH (1ST MONDAY)

Tuna sandwich on whole wheat, with lettuce and tomato (light mayo)
Crisp apple
Iced tea or seltzer with lemon

AFTERNOON STRESS RELEASE (1ST MONDAY)

Lie or sit comfortably and breathe in slowly through your nose. Visualize your breath as it enters your sinuses, flows down into your chest, and expands your rib cage. Slowly breathe out through your nose, following the breath as it rises through your chest and sinuses, and finally leaves your body. Repeat slowly for 1 to 2 minutes.

AFTERNOON SNACK (1ST MONDAY)

1 cup tomato soup or juice
1 to 2 ounces (up to ¼ cup) of unsalted almonds or walnuts
Iced tea or water with lemon

AFTERNOON MENTAL AEROBICS (1ST MONDAY)

Write down the two details that you committed to memory before leaving the house this morning. Check the piece of paper in your wallet to see how you did.

DINNER (1ST MONDAY)

Tossed green salad with balsamic vinegar and olive oil dressing
Grilled 6-ounce chicken breast with herbs
½ cup brown rice
Steamed spinach
Fruit sorbet
Seltzer, decaf iced tea, water, and/or a glass of wine

EVENING FITNESS/STRESS RELEASE (1ST MONDAY)

10-minute after-dinner walk, followed by a glass of water.
If circumstances do not permit a walk, repeat this morning's **Wake-Up Stretch and Conditioning** routine.

EVENING MENTAL AEROBICS (1ST MONDAY)

What number follows next in this sequence?

$$4 \quad 9 \quad 16 \quad 25 \quad \underline{\hspace{3cm}}$$

(Answer at end of 14-Day Prescription)

NIGHTTIME SNACK (1ST MONDAY)

Banana

OR

Frozen banana/peanut-butter sandwich: ½ banana sliced length-wise, spread
1 teaspoon natural peanut butter (low sugar) in middle, wrap in tin foil
and freeze.

1ST TUESDAY (DAY TWO)

*Tip for the Day: A brisk walk is known the world over as a great way to begin or
end a productive day. Start slowly, and pick up the pace as you go. Be sure to
gently stretch your muscles before and after your walk.*

WAKE-UP STRETCH AND CONDITIONING (1ST TUESDAY)

Stretch #1 [*Deep Breathing Dips*] (See 1st Monday)

Stretch #2 [*Side Stretch*] Stand with feet forward and shoulder width apart,
knees slightly bent. Raise your right hand overhead and lean over to your left
side. Reach as far to the left as you can, then hold and breathe for a count of
five. Slowly bring your torso upright while exhaling. Raise your left arm overhead, reaching to the right side as far as you can. Hold and breathe for a
count of five. Slowly return to upright. Repeat both sides.

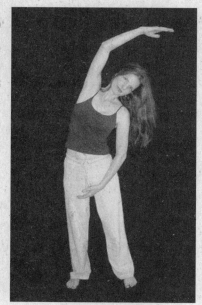

Side Stretch

Conditioning Exercise #1 [*Russian Dancer Knee Lifts*] Repeat for a count of **20**. (See 1st Monday)

Drink a glass of water.

BREAKFAST (1ST TUESDAY)

¾ cup hot oatmeal with 1 tablespoon raisins
½ cup nonfat milk or yogurt
½ grapefruit
Tea, coffee, water, or sparkling juice
Daily vitamin supplements: 1 multivitamin; vitamin C—500 mgs; vitamin
    E—400 IUs; omega-3 fatty acid—1,000 mgs

FITNESS ON THE RUN (1ST TUESDAY)

Park or get dropped off at a distance from your first destination of the day and walk briskly the rest of the way.

OR: **5-minute** morning walk.

Skip the elevator and take the stairs.

Drink a glass of water.

MORNING MENTAL AEROBICS (1ST TUESDAY)

Try to learn the following list of words by concentrating and repeating them out loud at least 5 times:

FLAG, DUNE, CARD, HEART, FENCE

MID-MORNING SNACK (1ST TUESDAY)

Hard-boiled egg (or 3 hard-boiled egg whites)
1 cup tomato soup or juice
Green tea or water

MID-MORNING MENTAL AEROBICS (1ST TUESDAY)

Get a paper and pencil. Using your left hand if you are right-handed, or vice-versa, draw the most perfect circle you can. Now shade it in fully, trying not to draw outside the line of the circle. When finished, sign your name to your masterpiece still using that opposite hand.

LUNCH (1ST TUESDAY)

Garden salad with 3 to 6 ounces grilled chicken and vinaigrette dressing
2 whole-grain crackers
Sliced pear
Iced tea or seltzer with lemon

AFTERNOON STRESS RELEASE (1ST TUESDAY)

Sit comfortably and imagine yourself at a beautiful beach just before sundown. Breathe deeply and rhythmically as you conjure up the details of the setting. Feel the misty ocean breeze. Hear the seagulls and the waves. Watch as the sun touches the horizon and begins to slip below it, bit by bit—now half, three-quarters, almost gone, and finally completely disappeared. Take one more deep breath, close your eyes, and exhale slowly. Open your eyes before continuing with your day.

AFTERNOON SNACK (1ST TUESDAY)

1 cup yogurt (frozen is fine)
½ cup blueberries
Iced tea or water with lemon

AFTERNOON MENTAL AEROBICS (1ST TUESDAY)

Do you remember the five words you repeated aloud this morning? If not, go back and try to memorize them again—but this time create a visual image for each word. Then, think of a little story to connect them.

DINNER (1ST TUESDAY)

Tomato, avocado, and sweet onion salad, with olive oil and vinegar
4 to 6 ounce grilled salmon filet with herbs and lemon slices

Boiled red potatoes

Steamed broccoli

Sliced fresh apple with cinnamon OR Cinnamon Baked Apple* [*see recipe, Appendix 2]

Seltzer, decaf iced tea, water, and/or a glass of wine

EVENING FITNESS/STRESS RELEASE (1ST TUESDAY)

10 to 15 minute after-dinner walk, or repeat this morning's Wake-Up Stretch and Conditioning routine.

Drink a glass of water.

EVENING MENTAL AEROBICS (1ST TUESDAY)

Here are a couple of brainteasers that might stump you:

(1) Which of the following words spelled backward is the odd one out?

DNALGNE   YLATI   SIRAP   ADANAC

(2) Question: John is standing behind Jim, but Jim is standing behind John. How can that be? (Answer at end of program)

NIGHTTIME SNACK (1ST TUESDAY)

Frozen fruit or fruit-juice bar

1ST WEDNESDAY (DAY THREE)

Tip for the Day: Drinking eight glasses of water a day is an important goal of the 14-Day Plan. Placing bottled water in handy places — car, desk, briefcase, etc. — makes it easier to keep drinking.

WAKE-UP STRETCH AND CONDITIONING (1ST WEDNESDAY)

Stretch #1 [*Deep Breathing Dips*]

Stretch #2 [*Side Stretch*] (See 1st Tuesday)

Conditioning Exercise #1 [*Russian Dancer Knee Lifts*] for a count of **30**.

Drink a glass of water.

BREAKFAST (1ST WEDNESDAY)

Scrambled eggs (2 egg whites plus one egg) with 2 strips turkey bacon
1 slice sourdough or rye toast with natural fruit jam
½ cup fresh or frozen blueberries
Tea, coffee, water, or sparkling juice
Vitamin supplements

MORNING MENTAL AEROBICS (1ST WEDNESDAY)

For each of the following four objects, create a vivid, detailed, and personally meaningful visual image: DOLL, SAILBOAT, BUILDING, OFFICE SUPPLY. Connect these images by creating a story that links them sequentially.

FITNESS ON THE RUN (1ST WEDNESDAY)

Park or get dropped off at a distance from your first destination of the day and walk briskly the rest of the way.

OR: **5-minute** morning walk.

Skip the elevator and take the stairs.

Drink a glass of water when you arrive.

MID-MORNING SNACK (1ST WEDNESDAY)

½ cup low-fat cottage cheese, plus 1 tablespoon raisins mixed in
½ banana
Green tea or water

MID-MORNING MENTAL AEROBICS (1ST WEDNESDAY)

The following proverb has had all of the vowels taken out and the remaining letters broken up into random groupings. Replace the vowels and find the proverb:

PPLW   HLV   NGLS   SHSS   SHLDNT   THR   WSTNS

LUNCH (1ST WEDNESDAY)

Bowl of chicken soup (with white meat and vegetables)
½ toasted pita bread
Orange sections
Iced tea or seltzer with lemon

AFTERNOON STRESS RELEASE (1ST WEDNESDAY)

Lie or sit comfortably. Take a deep breath and let it out slowly. Focus attention on your head and scalp and imagine releasing all the tension there. Move your focus down to your facial muscles, releasing any tension there. Let the relaxed feeling extend through your cheeks and jaw, down your neck and into your shoulders, releasing tension while breathing slowly and deeply. Continue down through your arms, hands, abdomen, back, hips, legs, feet, and toes—releasing all tension. Keep breathing deeply for 1 to 3 minutes, allowing every last bit of tension to leave your body as you exhale. When possible, do this exercise with your eyes closed.

AFTERNOON SNACK (1ST WEDNESDAY)

Bag of raw vegetables: celery/red bell pepper/tomatoes
1 ounce string cheese
Iced tea or water with lemon

AFTERNOON MENTAL AEROBICS (1ST WEDNESDAY)

Attempt to remember the four objects you memorized this morning. Try to recall the story you created that linked the images.

DINNER (1ST WEDNESDAY)

Spinach salad with chopped apple and walnuts, with vinaigrette dressing
Turkey burger on toasted whole wheat OR Turkey and Veggie Chili* (save
     leftovers for tomorrow's lunch)
Steamed spinach and carrots
Peach slices topped with vanilla yogurt and a tablespoon of chopped wal-
     nuts
Seltzer, decaf iced tea, water, and/or a glass of wine

EVENING FITNESS/STRESS RELEASE (1ST WEDNESDAY)

10 to 15 minute after-dinner walk, or repeat this morning's Wake-Up Stretch and Conditioning routine.

Drink a glass of water.

EVENING MENTAL AEROBICS (1ST WEDNESDAY)

Elaborating visual detail helps us create more memorable visual images. Try the following elaboration exercises:

1. Sit in a comfortable chair, close your eyes, and think of the first thing that comes to mind, be it an object, situation, person, or animal. Now try to imagine greater detail about how it looks or feels.

2. For each of the following, create a colorful, vivid, and detailed visual image (e.g., rather than just a dog, visualize a salivating brown dachshund with a muddy coat):

   - **car**
   - **hat**
   - **athlete**

NIGHTTIME SNACK (1ST WEDNESDAY)

Frozen yogurt

1ST THURSDAY (DAY FOUR)

Tip for the Day: We often don't remember life's details because we don't pay attention long enough to learn new information. Make a conscious effort to focus on one thing you might not otherwise notice—such as something a family member or friend has scheduled today. Ask them about it this evening and watch their response.

WAKE-UP STRETCH AND CONDITIONING (1ST THURSDAY)

Stretch #1 [*Deep Breathing Dips*]

Stretch #2 [*Side Stretch*]

Conditioning Exercise #1 [*Russian Dancer Knee Lifts*] for a count of **30**.

Conditioning Exercise #2: [*Marching Soldier*] Stand upright and march in place, lifting your knees waist-high. With each step, swing your straight arms forward and back, as far and high as possible, getting a good rotation in the shoulder. Continue marching for a count of **20**.

Drink a glass of water.

BREAKFAST (1ST THURSDAY)

Breakfast burrito (3 egg whites scrambled with 1 ounce shredded cheddar cheese plus 1 tablespoon salsa; roll in warmed corn tortilla)
Orange sections
Tea, coffee, water, or sparkling juice
Vitamin supplements

MORNING MENTAL AEROBICS (1ST THURSDAY)

During this first week, you are beginning to familiarize yourself with the three skills basic to all memory techniques: *LOOK, SNAP,* and *CONNECT:*

1. LOOK: Actively observe what you wish to remember. Take your time, focus, and concentrate. *LOOK* stands for all five senses—listen, smell, feel, and taste also contribute to effective learning.

2. SNAP: Create a mental snapshot, since most people find it much easier to learn and recall visual images than any other kind of information.

3. CONNECT: Link up your visual images or *SNAPs* for later re-call.

Many of the mental aerobics exercises will teach you to apply these skills effectively so you can use them in practical everyday situations. To help you develop your ability to use CONNECT, imagine a logical connection between each of the following word pairs:

Telephone — Sink

Hammer — Stuffed Animal

Orange — Fireman

Wig — Basketball

[For a more detailed explanation of LOOK, SNAP, CONNECT, see Chapter 6.]

FITNESS ON THE RUN (1ST THURSDAY)

Park or get dropped off at a distance from your first destination of the day and walk briskly the rest of the way.

OR: **10-minute** morning walk.

Skip the elevator and take the stairs.

Drink a glass of water.

MID-MORNING SNACK (1ST THURSDAY)

3/4 cup yogurt with sliced banana OR Banana/Strawberry Yogurt Smoothie*

MID-MORNING MENTAL AEROBICS (1ST THURSDAY)

Go back to the word pairs you worked on earlier and now imagine a bizarre or illogical connection for each. For example, instead of imagining the telephone placed next to the sink, visualize the telephone washing down the drain of the sink.

49

> *Telephone — Sink*
> *Hammer — Stuffed Animal*
> *Orange — Fireman*
> *Wig — Basketball*

LUNCH (1ST THURSDAY)

Sliced roast beef sandwich on rye OR leftover Turkey and Veggie Chili* and
    2 bread sticks
Celery and carrot slices
Iced tea or seltzer with lemon

AFTERNOON STRESS RELEASE (1ST THURSDAY)

Lie down or sit comfortably and breathe in slowly through your nose. Visualize your breath as it enters your sinuses, flows down into your chest, and expands your rib cage. Slowly breathe out through your nose, following the breath as it rises through your chest and sinuses, and finally leaves your body. Repeat slowly for 1 to 2 minutes.

AFTERNOON SNACK (1ST THURSDAY)

1 cup tomato soup or juice
1 to 2 ounces (up to ¼ cup) of unsalted walnuts or almonds
Iced tea or water with lemon

AFTERNOON MENTAL AEROBICS (1ST THURSDAY)

Many names are easy to remember because they bring a mental image to mind. Mr. Lincoln makes me think of Lincoln Monument. Mrs. Katz brings up an image of cats. For other names we can create substitute images. For Bill, think of a dollar bill. Conjure up a visual image for each of the following names — often your first association will be the most effective one. Sometimes an association to someone famous or someone you know well will help. Also try substituting easily visualized words that sound like the name.

> *Frank*
> *Dinah*
> *Mike*
> *Simon*
> *Barbara*
> *Jim*
> *Phillip*
> *George*

(Take a look at some possible answers at the end of the program only after you have made a few attempts at this exercise.)

DINNER (1ST THURSDAY)

Tomato, avocado, and sweet onion salad, with olive oil and vinegar
Broiled 4 to 6 ounce halibut with salsa
½ cup brown rice
Steamed broccoli
Fruit sorbet OR Pear Crisp*
Seltzer, decaf iced tea, water, and/or a glass of wine

EVENING FITNESS STRESS RELEASE (1ST THURSDAY)

10 to 15 minute after-dinner walk.

OR: repeat this morning's Wake-Up Stretch and Conditioning routine.

Drink a glass of water.

EVENING MENTAL AEROBICS (1ST THURSDAY)

Practice your mental organizational skills. Group the following 12 items into 3 categories:

Pool	Punch line	Facsimile
Memo	Pond	Jibe
Pun	Lagoon	IOU
Lake	Post-it	Gag

Now that you are mentally sharp from your organization exercise, try to recall the mental snapshots you conjured up this afternoon for several names. How many of them do you recall?

NIGHTTIME SNACK (1ST THURSDAY)

Red or green grapes

1ST FRIDAY (DAY FIVE)

Tip for the Day: Remembering names and faces is THE number one memory complaint. The next time you meet someone new, try these techniques to help to remember their name:

- Repeat the person's name during your conversation
- Comment if the person reminds you of someone else you know
- If appropriate, ask the person to spell their name or pronounce it slowly
- Use the name when you say good-bye

WAKE-UP STRETCH AND CONDITIONING (1ST FRIDAY)

Stretch #1 [*Deep Breathing Dips*]

Stretch #3 [*Chest/Back Expanders*] Stand with feet shoulder width apart, interlace your fingers with palms away from your body, and push your arms straight out in front of you as far as you can (Figure 1). Hold for 2 to 4 seconds, release, and repeat. Now link your hands behind your back. Lift them up slightly, pushing them back and away from your body (Figure 2). Hold for 2 to 4 seconds, release, and repeat. (If it is difficult to link your hands behind your back, stretch a rolled towel between them and grab the towel.)

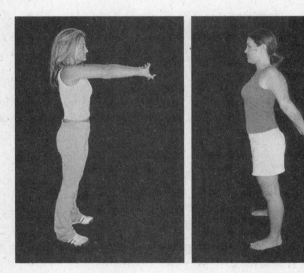

Figure 1   Figure 2

Chest/Back Expansion

Conditioning Exercise #1 [*Russian Dancer Knee Lifts*] for a count of 40.

Conditioning Exercise #2 [*Marching Soldier*] for a count of **20**. (See 1st Thursday)

Drink a glass of water.

BREAKFAST (1ST FRIDAY)

Whole wheat French toast (use 1 egg plus 1 egg white) served with natural
    fruit jam OR Orange Grove French Toast*
½ cup low-fat cottage cheese with ½ cup fresh or frozen blueberries
Tea, coffee, water, or sparkling juice
Vitamin supplements

MORNING MENTAL AEROBICS (1ST FRIDAY)

Use *LOOK* (actively observe what you wish to remember), *SNAP* (create a mental snapshot of the information to remember), *CONNECT* (link up your visual snapshots) to learn and associate together the following unrelated word pairs.

> *Texas — glass*
> *Moon — washer*
> *Blouse — hose*
> *Novel — broccoli*
> *Cloud — wrench*

FITNESS ON THE RUN (1ST FRIDAY)

Park or get dropped off at a distance from your first destination of the day and walk briskly the rest of the way.

OR: **10-minute** morning walk.

Skip the elevator and take the stairs.

Drink a glass of water.

MID-MORNING SNACK (1ST FRIDAY)

1 cup chicken soup
½ apple sliced, sprinkled with cinnamon
Green tea or water

MID-MORNING MENTAL AEROBICS (1ST FRIDAY)

Elaborating detail will help you create mental SNAPs that stay fixed in memory. For each of the following objects, think of three details you can visualize:

Tomato

Glove

Watch

Car

Flower

LUNCH (1ST FRIDAY)

Garden vegetable salad with chicken and vinaigrette dressing
Iced tea or seltzer with lemon

AFTERNOON STRESS RELEASE (1ST FRIDAY)

Sit comfortably and imagine yourself at a beautiful beach just before sundown. Breathe deeply and rhythmically as you conjure up the details of the setting. Feel the misty ocean breeze. Hear the seagulls and the waves. Watch as the sun touches the horizon and begins to slip below it, bit by bit—now half, three-quarters, almost gone, and finally completely disappeared. Take one more deep breath, close your eyes, and exhale slowly. Open your eyes before continuing with your day.

AFTERNOON SNACK (1ST FRIDAY)

½ cup yogurt, plus 1 tablespoon raisins mixed in, OR Peanut Butter/
  Ricotta Spread* on celery sticks
Peach or pear
Iced tea or water with lemon

AFTERNOON MENTAL AEROBICS (1ST FRIDAY)

Let's see if *LOOK, SNAP, CONNECT* helped you remember this morning's word pairs. Here is the first word; see if you recall the second word:

Texas — _____
Moon — _____
Blouse — _____
Novel — _____
Cloud — _____

DINNER (1ST FRIDAY)

Tomato, avocado, and sweet onion salad drizzled with olive oil and
  vinegar
Grilled 4 to 6 ounce salmon steak with herbs
Steamed Brussels sprouts
½ cup brown rice OR Wild Rice*
Frozen fruit or fruit juice bar OR Featherweight Cheesecake*
Seltzer, decaf iced tea, water, and/or a glass of wine

EVENING FITNESS/STRESS RELEASE (1ST FRIDAY)

10 to 15 minute after-dinner walk, or repeat this morning's Wake-Up Stretch and Conditioning routine.

Drink a glass of water.

EVENING MENTAL AEROBICS (1ST FRIDAY)

This morning, you did an elaboration exercise, thinking of at least four details that you could visualize for each object. Can you remember the objects? Can you still see the four details?

NIGHTTIME SNACK (1ST FRIDAY)

Banana
OR
Frozen banana/peanut-butter sandwich: ½ banana sliced lengthwise, spread 1 teaspoon peanut butter in middle, wrap in tin foil and freeze.

1ST SATURDAY (DAY SIX)

Tip for the Day: The most common cause of lost time at work is backache. Back trouble is often the result of chronic tension. Try to stretch your back and chest muscles every day to release stored tension and allow for increased strengthening.

WAKE-UP STRETCH AND CONDITIONING (1ST SATURDAY)

Stretch #1 [*Deep Breathing Dips*]

Stretch #2 [*Side Stretch*]

Stretch #3 [*Chest/Back Expanders*] (See 1st Friday)

Conditioning Exercise #1 [*Russian Dancer Knee Lifts*] for a count of **40**.

Conditioning Exercise #2 [*Marching Soldier*] for a count of **20**.

Drink a glass of water.

BREAKFAST (1ST SATURDAY)

Open-face egg-white sandwich (2 cooked egg whites on 1 slice sourdough
    toast with 1 ounce cheddar cheese and tomato or natural jam)
Fresh orange or pineapple slices
Tea, coffee, water, or sparkling juice
Vitamin supplements

MORNING MENTAL AEROBICS (1ST SATURDAY)

Practice your mental organizational skills. Group the following 12 items into
3 categories:

Yarn	Drawer	Vial
Tobacco tin	Suture	Lentil
Pepper	Shoebox	Wick
Cocoa	Licorice	Dental floss

This kind of exercise can be useful for remembering lists of items at the store.
Placing them in categories helps organize the shopping trip (you think of all
the vegetables you need when you're in that section of the store). After your
first attempts, check the answer at the end of the program.

WEEKEND FITNESS (1ST SATURDAY)

13 to 30 minute morning walk.

OR: Treadmill, bicycle, workout of your choice.

Drink a glass of water.

MID-MORNING SNACK (1ST SATURDAY)

½ apple, sliced
½ cup low-fat cottage cheese OR Peanut Butter/Ricotta Spread*
Green tea or water

MID-MORNING MENTAL AEROBICS (1ST SATURDAY)

When we are stress-free, we are better at concentrating and learning. Before you begin this mental aerobics exercise, take a **one-minute stress-release break:** Breathe in and out slowly through your nose. Follow your breath as it rises through your chest and sinuses, and finally leaves your body. Repeat slowly for one minute.

Now that you are relaxed, create a single visual image to link each of the following groups of words. After you create the visual images, try to see them in your mind's eye and connect them together to help you memorize them. To help connect the SNAPs, include action in them, merge or penetrate the SNAPs, or place them next to each other. For example, visualize the lion with a toothpick in its mouth.

> *Toothpick — lion — rose bush*
> *Computer — potato — scooter*
> *Palm tree — bull — blimp*
> *Parachute — thumb — apple*

LUNCH (1ST SATURDAY)

Grilled turkey-dog on rye toast with mustard (sauerkraut optional)
Grapes
Iced tea or seltzer with lemon

AFTERNOON STRESS RELEASE (1ST SATURDAY)

Sit comfortably or lie down. If possible, do the following with your eyes closed: take a deep breath in, and then let it out slowly. Focus attention on your head and scalp and imagine releasing all the tension there. Bring your focus down to your facial muscles and release that tension. Let the relaxed feeling extend through your cheeks and jaw, down into your neck and shoulders, releasing the tension there while breathing in and out slowly and deeply. Continue moving systematically down your body through your arms, hands, abdomen, back, hips, legs, and toes. Continue to breathe deeply for 1 to 3 minutes allowing even more tension to leave your body with each exhalation.

AFTERNOON SNACK (1ST SATURDAY)

Sliced raw vegetables
String cheese OR Hummus Dip*
Iced tea or water with lemon

AFTERNOON MENTAL AEROBICS (1ST SATURDAY)

Begin with your one-minute stress release (see Mid-Morning Mental Aerobics). Try to recall the images from your last mental aerobics exercise. If you can't recall them from scratch, use the first words to jog your memory of the other words (remember to conjure up the connecting mental snapshots you created).

If you need them, here are the first words:

Toothpick . . .
Computer . . .
Palm tree . . .
Parachute . . .

DINNER (1ST SATURDAY)

Arugula and shaved Parmesan cheese salad tossed in balsamic vinegar and
  olive oil dressing
Sliced chicken breast with fettuccine and tomato sauce
Steamed zucchini rounds
Sliced strawberries (may be drizzled with 1 teaspoon chocolate sauce and
  chopped peanuts)
Seltzer, decaf iced tea, water, and/or a glass of wine

EVENING FITNESS/STRESS RELEASE (1ST SATURDAY)

10 to 15 minute after-dinner walk.

OR: repeat this morning's Wake-Up Stretch and Conditioning routine.

Drink a glass of water.

EVENING MENTAL AEROBICS (1ST SATURDAY)

Which letter or number is the odd one in each rectangle?

M	H	
R	X	
B	O	
	Q	

21	35		
16	9		26
	18	46	28

NIGHTTIME SNACK (1ST SATURDAY)

Popcorn (air-pop or microwave, hold the butter)

1ST SUNDAY (DAY SEVEN)

Tip for the Day: Many of us react to stress by eating, often choosing foods that do not promote brain health. Take a few minutes today to make your home or office a more snack-friendly environment. Remove some unhealthy stress-snacks (e.g., cookies, chips, candy, etc.) and replace them with healthy brain food (e.g., fresh and/or dried fruits, rye croutons, whole grain baked crackers, sliced raw vegetables, rice cakes, etc.).

WAKE-UP STRETCH AND CONDITIONING (1ST SUNDAY)

Stretch #1 [*Deep Breathing Dips*]

Stretch #2 [*Side Stretch*]

Stretch #3 [*Chest/Back Expander*]

Conditioning Exercise #2 [*Marching Soldier*] for a count of **30**.

Conditioning Exercise #3 [*Standing Crunches*] Stand straight with feet slightly apart. Lift your arms straight overhead, palms facing each other, and hands fisted (Figure 1). Take a deep breath in. Exhale as you lift your right knee and pull your arms down powerfully, as if there were weights in your fists, bending at the elbow (Figure 2). Breathe in as your arms go back up, and repeat with left knee. Keep your stomach pulled in and tight, especially as you exhale, lift your knee and pull your arms down. Repeat for a total count of **20**.

Drink a glass of water.

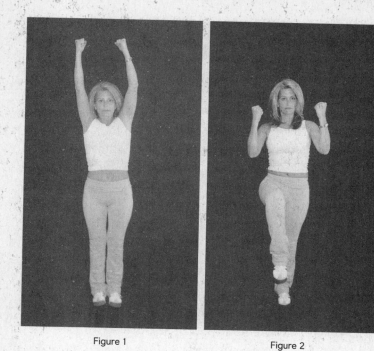

Figure 1   Figure 2

Standing Crunches

BREAKFAST (1ST SUNDAY)

Toasted onion bagel served with low-fat cream cheese and 1 slice smoked
    salmon, add tomato and onion as desired
Mixed berries
Tea, coffee, water, or sparkling juice
Vitamin supplements

MORNING MENTAL AEROBICS (1ST SUNDAY)

Before leaving the house, think of three errands or tasks you need to accomplish today. Create a *SNAP* or visual image for each and then *CONNECT*

them together in the order you plan to do them. Take your time and really let the images sink in.

WEEKEND FITNESS (1ST SUNDAY)

15 to 30 minute morning walk.

OR: Treadmill, bicycle, workout of your choice.

Drink a glass of water.

MID-MORNING SNACK (1ST SUNDAY)

Hard-boiled egg (or 3 egg whites)
1 cup vegetable soup of choice
Green tea or water

MID-MORNING MENTAL AEROBICS (1ST SUNDAY)

Begin with your one-minute stress release (see yesterday's Mid-Morning Mental Aerobics).

Learning and remembering complex names that do not bring to mind a mental image can be a challenge. For those names or the syllables and sounds within them, we can substitute names or sounds that do have a meaning. By linking these substitute words together, we can create a visual image that works. Weinkauf becomes wine-cough (see someone sipping wine and then coughing). To develop this skill, create a SNAP for each of the following names (use substitutes to conjure up an image for each syllable and then CONNECT them):

> *Maremont*
> *Laghrissi*
> *Marseille*

(See end of 14-Day Plan for possible answers.)

LUNCH (1ST SUNDAY)

Salad Niçoise (butter lettuce with tuna, green beans, tomatoes, olives, egg
    whites, red pepper, and artichoke hearts, tossed in olive oil and vinegar
    dressing)
Iced tea or seltzer with lemon

AFTERNOON STRESS RELEASE (1ST SUNDAY)

Lie down or sit comfortably and breathe in slowly through your nose. Visualize your breath as it enters your sinuses, flows down into your chest, and expands your rib cage. Slowly breathe out through your nose, following the
breath as it rises through your chest and sinuses, and finally leaves your body.
Repeat slowly for 1 to 2 minutes.

AFTERNOON SNACK (1ST SUNDAY)

Guacamole (mashed avocado, 2 tablespoons plain yogurt, 1/4 cup drained
    salsa, and lemon juice to taste)
Sliced fresh vegetables OR Baked Corn Tortilla Chips*
Iced tea or water with lemon

AFTERNOON MENTAL AEROBICS (1ST SUNDAY)

Begin with your one-minute stress release. Fine tune your observation skills
(LOOK) to improve your ability to remember faces. Focus on some distinguishing feature or detail that you notice on the faces of the next two people
you see this afternoon.

DINNER (1ST SUNDAY)

Spinach salad with chopped apple and walnuts, red wine vinegar and olive
   oil
4 to 6 ounce grilled sirloin steak (or chicken)
½ of a baked potato topped with chives OR corn-on-the-cob
Frozen yogurt OR Cinnamon Baked Apple*
Seltzer, decaf iced tea, water, and/or a glass of wine

EVENING FITNESS/STRESS RELEASE (1ST SUNDAY)

10 to 15 minute after-dinner walk.

OR: repeat this morning's Wake-Up Stretch and Conditioning routine.

Drink a glass of water.

EVENING MENTAL AEROBICS (1ST SUNDAY)

Do you recall the distinguishing facial features of the people you saw this afternoon? Did you remember to carry out your three errands from the morning?

NIGHTTIME SNACK (1ST SUNDAY)

Fresh or frozen mixed berries

Congratulations! You have completed your first week of the 14-Day Plan. You should be feeling a higher level of energy and mental capacity. In the next seven days your new lifestyle habits will take hold and not only will you notice changes in your health and appearance, but so will those around you. Carry on.

2ND MONDAY (DAY EIGHT)

Tip for the Day: Almost everyone forgets where they put their keys or glasses on occasion. To help avoid misplacing commonly used items, create "memory places"— a drawer or hook in the kitchen for your car keys, a specific "memory shelf" for your glasses, a utility drawer in the desk for scissors, pencils, and tape, etc.

WAKE-UP STRETCH AND CONDITIONING (2ND MONDAY)

Stretch #1 [*Deep Breathing Dips*]

Stretch #2 [*Side Stretch*]

Stretch #3 [*Chest/Back Expander*]

Conditioning Exercise #1 [*Russian Dancer Knee Lifts*] for a count of **40**.

Conditioning Exercise #3 [*Standing Crunches*] (See 1st Sunday) for a count of **20**.

Drink a glass of water.

BREAKFAST (2ND MONDAY)

Vegetable omelet (use 1 whole egg plus 2 egg whites)
½ cup fresh or frozen blueberries
Tea, coffee, water, or sparkling juice
Vitamin supplements

MORNING MENTAL AEROBICS (2ND MONDAY)

Brush up on *LOOK, SNAP, CONNECT*. Memorize the following word pairs for recall later:

Ship—Bulb
Tomato—Saddle
Caterpillar—Artichoke
Teacher—Soap
Slipper—Pool
Daisy—Lightning
Engine—Wine

FITNESS ON THE RUN (2ND MONDAY)

Park or get dropped off at a distance from your first destination of the day and walk briskly the rest of the way.

OR: **15-minute** morning walk.

Skip the elevator and take the stairs.

Drink a glass of water.

MID-MORNING SNACK (2ND MONDAY)

½ cup nonfat plain or flavored yogurt with 1 tablespoon raisins
Green tea or water

MID-MORNING MENTAL AEROBICS (2ND MONDAY)

Begin with your one-minute stress release.

Here are the first words for the word pairs you learned earlier today. See how many of the pairs you recall:

*Ship—*_____
*Tomato—*_____

Caterpillar—_____
Teacher—_____
Slipper—_____
Daisy—_____
Engine—_____

LUNCH (2ND MONDAY)

Tuna sandwich on whole wheat, with lettuce and tomato (light mayo)
Crisp apple
Iced tea or seltzer with lemon

AFTERNOON STRESS RELEASE (2ND MONDAY)

Sit comfortably and imagine yourself at a beautiful beach just before sundown. Breathe deeply and rhythmically as you conjure up the details of the setting. Feel the misty ocean breeze. Hear the seagulls and the waves. Watch as the sun touches the horizon and begins to slip below it, bit by bit—now half, three-quarters, almost gone, and finally completely disappeared. Take one more deep breath, close your eyes, and exhale slowly. Open your eyes before continuing with your day.

AFTERNOON SNACK (2ND MONDAY)

1 cup tomato soup or juice
1 to 2 ounces (up to ¼ cup) of unsalted almonds or walnuts
Iced tea or water with lemon

AFTERNOON MENTAL AEROBICS (2ND MONDAY)

Your mate or friend reminds you that you will be meeting Paul Foreman at the reception this evening. Use *SNAP* and *CONNECT* to create a mental image to represent his name.

(If you need help, see a suggested approach at the end of the program.)

DINNER (2ND MONDAY)

Tossed green salad with balsamic vinegar and olive oil dressing
Grilled 4 to 6 ounce chicken breast with herbs OR Chicken Cacciatore*
½ cup brown rice OR fettuccini with fresh basil
Steamed zucchini
Fruit sorbet
Seltzer, decaf iced tea, water, and/or a glass of wine

EVENING FITNESS/STRESS RELEASE (2ND MONDAY)

10 to 15 minute after-dinner walk, or repeat this morning's Wake-Up Stretch and Conditioning routine.

Drink a glass of water.

EVENING MENTAL AEROBICS (2ND MONDAY)

You now have the delight of meeting Paul Foreman. You have already created a *SNAP* for his name. Now focus on his face below, notice a distinguishing

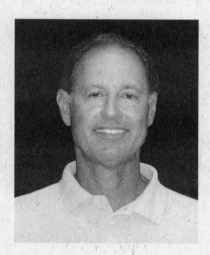

feature, create a *SNAP* for it, and *CONNECT* the "face" *SNAP* with the "name" *SNAP*.

NIGHTTIME SNACK (2ND MONDAY)

Banana

OR

Frozen banana/peanut-butter sandwich (see 1st Monday Nighttime Snack)

2ND TUESDAY (DAY NINE)

Tip for the Day: Keeping your muscles stretched and limber helps protect you from common injuries. Lightly stretching your thighs, hamstrings, calves, and shoulders after your walk or workout will help keep your muscles loose and your movement fluid.

WAKE-UP STRETCH AND CONDITIONING (2ND TUESDAY)

Stretch #1 [*Deep Breathing Dips*]

Stretch #2 [*Side Stretch*]

Stretch #3 [*Chest/Back Expander*]

Conditioning Exercise #2 [*Marching Soldier*] for a count of 30.

Conditioning Exercise #3 [*Standing Crunches*] for a count of 20.

Drink a glass of water.

BREAKFAST (2ND TUESDAY)

¾ cup hot oatmeal with 1 tablespoon raisins
½ cup nonfat milk or yogurt
½ grapefruit
Tea, coffee, water, or sparkling juice
Vitamin supplements

MORNING MENTAL AEROBICS (2ND TUESDAY)

For each of the following four objects, create a vivid, detailed, and personally meaningful visual image. Connect these images by creating a story that links them sequentially.

Athlete
Animal
Drink
Antique

FITNESS ON THE RUN (2ND TUESDAY)

Park or get dropped off at a distance from your first destination of the day and walk briskly the rest of the way.

OR: **15-minute** morning walk.

Skip the elevator and take the stairs.

Drink a glass of water.

MID-MORNING SNACK (2ND TUESDAY)

Hard-boiled egg (or 3 hard-boiled egg whites)
1 cup tomato soup or juice
Green tea or water

MID-MORNING MENTAL AEROBICS (2ND TUESDAY)

Try this paper and pencil exercise once again. Using your left hand if you are right-handed, or vice-versa, draw the most perfect circle you can. Now pencil it in fully, trying not to draw outside the line of the circle. Still using that opposite hand, use scissors to cut out the circle.

LUNCH (2ND TUESDAY)

Garden salad with grilled chicken and vinaigrette dressing
2 whole grain crackers
Sliced pear
Iced tea or seltzer with lemon

AFTERNOON STRESS RELEASE (2ND TUESDAY)

Sit comfortably or lie down. If possible, do the following with your eyes closed: take a deep breath in, and then let it out slowly. Focus attention on your head and scalp and imagine releasing all the tension there. Bring your focus down to your facial muscles and release that tension. Let the relaxed feeling extend through your cheeks and jaw, down into your neck and shoulders, releasing the tension there while breathing in and out slowly and deeply. Continue moving systematically down your body through your arms, hands, abdomen, back, hips, legs, and toes. Continue to breathe deeply for 1 to 3 minutes, allowing more tension to leave your body with each exhale.

AFTERNOON SNACK (2ND TUESDAY)

1 cup yogurt
½ cup blueberries
Iced tea or water with lemon

AFTERNOON MENTAL AEROBICS (2ND TUESDAY)

See if you can remember the four objects you memorized this morning. Try to recall the story you created that linked the images.

DINNER (2ND TUESDAY)

Tomato, avocado, and sweet onion salad, with olive oil and vinegar
Grilled 4 to 6 ounce salmon filet with herbs and lemon slices
Boiled red potatoes
Steamed broccoli
Sliced fresh apple with cinnamon OR Cinnamon Baked Apple*
Seltzer, decaf iced tea, water, and/or a glass of wine

EVENING FITNESS/STRESS RELEASE (2ND TUESDAY)

10 to 15 minute after-dinner walk.

OR: repeat this morning's Wake-Up Stretch and Conditioning routine.

Drink a glass of water.

EVENING MENTAL AEROBICS (2ND TUESDAY)

At the end of your evening walk, you see the familiar face below. What's his name again?

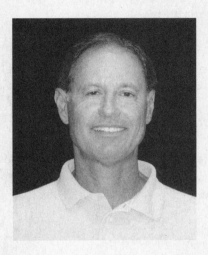

NIGHTTIME SNACK (2ND TUESDAY)

Frozen fruit or fruit-juice bar

2ND WEDNESDAY (DAY TEN)

Tip for the Day: Relaxation breaks or stress releases are wonderful breathers for your mind and body. Remember that with the 14-Day Plan, you are "training" yourself to relax, and like any skill, it requires practice. Allow yourself time to develop the techniques in order to achieve optimal results. (See Chapter 8 for more stress release suggestions.)

WAKE-UP STRETCH AND CONDITIONING (2ND WEDNESDAY)

Stretch #1 [*Deep Breathing Dips*]

Stretch #2 [*Side Stretch*]

Stretch #3 [*Chest/Back Expander*]

Conditioning Exercise #1 [*Russian Dancer Knee Lifts*] for a count of **40**.

Conditioning Exercise #2 [*Marching Soldier*] for a count of **30**.

Conditioning Exercise #3 [*Standing Crunches*] for a count of **20**.

Drink a glass of water.

BREAKFAST (2ND WEDNESDAY)

Scrambled eggs (3 egg whites) with 2 strips turkey bacon
1 slice sourdough or rye toast with natural fruit jam
½ cup fresh or frozen blueberries
Tea, coffee, water, or sparkling juice
Vitamin supplements

MORNING MENTAL AEROBICS (2ND WEDNESDAY)

Begin with your one-minute stress release.
Let's try to perfect the unrelated word-pair task, using *LOOK, SNAP, CON-NECT*. Here's a new list that I want you to memorize and recall later:

> *Tiger—Dresser*
> *Web—Chalkboard*
> *Screen—Island*

Scooter—Eagle
Toaster—Bubble
Scar—Shark
Garage—Sleet

FITNESS ON THE RUN (2ND WEDNESDAY)

Park or get dropped off at a distance from your first destination of the day and walk briskly the rest of the way.

OR: **15-minute** morning walk.

Skip the elevator and take the stairs.

Drink a glass of water.

MID-MORNING SNACK (2ND WEDNESDAY)

½ cup low-fat cottage cheese, with 1 tablespoon raisins mixed in
½ banana
Green tea or water

MID-MORNING MENTAL AEROBICS (2ND WEDNESDAY)

Begin with your one-minute stress release.

Let's see how you do on remembering the word pairs from this morning:

Tiger—_____
Web—_____
Screen—_____
Scooter—_____
Toaster—_____

*Scar—*_____
*Garage—*_____

LUNCH (2ND WEDNESDAY)

Bowl of chicken soup
½ toasted pita bread
Orange sections
Iced tea or seltzer with lemon

AFTERNOON STRESS RELEASE (2ND WEDNESDAY)

Lie down or sit comfortably and breathe in slowly through your nose. Visualize your breath as it enters your sinuses, flows down into your chest, and expands your rib cage. Slowly breathe out through your nose, following the breath as it rises through your chest and sinuses, and finally leaves your body. Repeat slowly for 1 to 2 minutes.

AFTERNOON SNACK (2ND WEDNESDAY)

Bag of raw vegetables: celery/red bell pepper/tomatoes
1 ounce string cheese
Iced tea or water with lemon

AFTERNOON MENTAL AEROBICS (2ND WEDNESDAY)

As quickly as you can, fill in the blank squares below so that the same words read across and down.

P	O	R	T
O			
R			
T			

DINNER (2ND WEDNESDAY)

Spinach salad with chopped apple and walnuts, and vinaigrette dressing
Turkey burger on whole wheat bun OR Turkey and Veggie Chili* (save left-
    overs for tomorrow's lunch)
Steamed spinach and carrots
Peach slices topped with vanilla yogurt and a tablespoon of chopped wal-
    nuts
Seltzer, decaf iced tea, water, and/or a glass of wine

EVENING FITNESS/STRESS RELEASE (2ND WEDNESDAY)

10 to 15 minute after-dinner walk, or repeat this morning's Wake-Up Stretch
and Conditioning routine.

Drink a glass of water.

EVENING MENTAL AEROBICS (2ND WEDNESDAY)

Which of the following shapes is different from the rest?

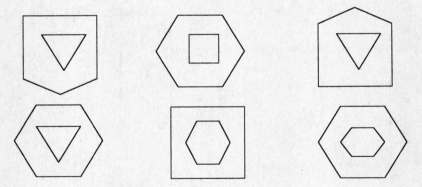

NIGHTTIME SNACK (2ND WEDNESDAY)

Frozen yogurt

2ND THURSDAY (DAY ELEVEN)

Tip for the Day: People who worry about their memory performance actually show poorer performance scores on memory tests compared to same-age non-worriers. Keep in mind that EVERYONE complains about memory loss with increasing age, even folks in their twenties and thirties. Minimizing undue worry about your memory may well improve it.

WAKE-UP STRETCH AND CONDITIONING (2ND THURSDAY)

Stretch #1 [*Deep Breathing Dips*]

Stretch #2 [*Side Stretch*]

Stretch #3 [*Chest/Back Expander*]

Conditioning Exercise #1 [*Russian Dancer Knee Lifts*] for a count of 50.

Conditioning Exercise #2 [*Marching Soldier*] for a count of 30.

Conditioning Exercise #3 [*Standing Crunches*] for a count of 20.

Drink a glass of water.

BREAKFAST (2ND THURSDAY)

Breakfast burrito (3 egg whites scrambled with 1 ounce shredded cheddar cheese plus 1 tablespoon salsa, rolled in warmed corn tortilla)
Orange sections

Tea, coffee, water, or sparkling juice
Vitamin supplements

MORNING MENTAL AEROBICS (2ND THURSDAY)

Creating SNAPs becomes more difficult when the word you want to remember is more abstract than concrete. "Theory" is harder to visualize than "surfboard." If you want to remember the word "theory," you might visualize "$E=mc^2$" written on a blackboard. Try your best to conjure up a visual image or SNAP for each of the following relatively abstract words (if needed, see the suggestions at the end of the program):

Social
Pressure
Outstanding
Hate

FITNESS ON THE RUN (2ND THURSDAY)

Park or get dropped off at a distance from your first destination of the day and walk briskly the rest of the way.

OR: **15-minute** morning walk.

Skip the elevator and take the stairs.

Drink a glass of water.

MID-MORNING SNACK (2ND THURSDAY)

¾ cup yogurt with sliced banana OR Banana/Strawberry Yogurt Smoothie*

MID-MORNING MENTAL AEROBICS (2ND THURSDAY)

Sometimes we hear a phone number that we only need to remember for a short while. This task can be made easier by *chunking* the numbers together in small groups and repeating the numbers until you make the call. Rather than remembering 3105558891, you think of three-ten (310), five-fifty-five (555), eighty-eight ninety-one (8891). If you recognize the area code, then that can be your starting point and you need not repeat it. Also, repeating it out loud makes it easier. Practice the technique on the following numbers or on three ten-digit phone numbers you actually use but do not know by heart:

416-853-1212
888-620-4183
212-555-2837

LUNCH (2ND THURSDAY)

Sliced roast beef sandwich on rye OR leftover Turkey and Veggie Chili* and
   2 bread sticks
Celery and carrot slices
Iced tea or seltzer with lemon

AFTERNOON STRESS RELEASE (2ND THURSDAY)

Sit comfortably and imagine yourself at a beautiful beach just before sundown. Breathe deeply and rhythmically as you conjure up the details of the setting. Feel the misty ocean breeze. Hear the seagulls and the waves. Watch as the sun touches the horizon and begins to slip below it, bit by bit—now half, three-quarters, almost gone, and finally completely disappeared. Take one more deep breath, close your eyes, and exhale slowly. Open your eyes before continuing with your day.

AFTERNOON SNACK (2ND THURSDAY)

1 cup tomato soup or juice
1 to 2 ounces (up to ¼ cup) of unsalted almonds or walnuts
Iced tea or water with lemon

AFTERNOON MENTAL AEROBICS (2ND THURSDAY)

Using the chunking method for remembering numbers, commit a frequently used, yet not memorized, phone number to memory. Take your time; break it up into three units: xxx, xxx, xxxx. Repeat it; say it aloud.

DINNER (2ND THURSDAY)

Tomato, avocado, and sweet onion salad, with olive oil and vinegar
Broiled 4 to 6 ounce halibut with salsa
½ cup brown rice
Steamed broccoli and cauliflower
Fruit sorbet OR Pear Crisp*
Seltzer, decaf iced tea, water, and/or a glass of wine

EVENING FITNESS/STRESS RELEASE (2ND THURSDAY)

10 to 15 minute after-dinner walk.

OR: repeat this morning's Wake-Up Stretch and Conditioning routine

Drink a glass of water.

EVENING MENTAL AEROBICS (2ND THURSDAY)

Do you remember the phone number you learned this afternoon? If so, try the technique with another phone number. If not, go back to the first one and practice again.

NIGHTTIME SNACK (2ND THURSDAY)

Red grapes

2ND FRIDAY (DAY TWELVE)

Tip for the Day: Chronic sleep deprivation can impair memory, concentration, and mood. Going to sleep 30 to 60 minutes earlier often helps people feel better. Twenty-minute daytime "power naps" can also be rejuvenating, but napping more than 30 minutes can leave you groggy when you wake.

WAKE-UP STRETCH AND CONDITIONING (2ND FRIDAY)

Stretch #1 [*Deep Breathing Dips*]

Stretch #2 [*Side Stretch*]

Stretch #3 [*Chest/Back Expander*]

Conditioning Exercise#1 [*Russian Dancer Knee Lifts*] for a count of **50**.

Conditioning Exercise #2 [*Marching Soldier*] for a count of **30**.

Conditioning Exercise #3 [*Standing Crunches*] for a count of **30**.

Drink a glass of water.

BREAKFAST (2ND FRIDAY)

¾ cup hot oatmeal with 1 tablespoon raisins OR Orange Grove French
    Toast*
½ cup low-fat cottage cheese
½ grapefruit

Tea, coffee, water, or sparkling juice
Vitamin supplements

MORNING MENTAL AEROBICS (2ND FRIDAY)

Begin with your **one-minute stress release**.

Now try the unrelated word-pair task with a list of words that may be a bit more challenging to visualize:

Architect—Idea
Legal—Eclipse
Future—Ornate
Outsider—Interpret
Clause—Shift

FITNESS ON THE RUN (2ND FRIDAY)

Park or get dropped off at a distance from your first destination of the day and walk briskly the rest of the way.

OR: **20-minute** morning walk.

Skip the elevator and take the stairs.

Drink a glass of water.

MID-MORNING SNACK (2ND FRIDAY)

1 cup chicken soup
½ apple sliced, sprinkled with cinnamon
Green tea or water

MID-MORNING MENTAL AEROBICS (2ND FRIDAY)

Begin with your **one-minute stress release**.

How many of the abstract word pairs can you recall?

Architect — _____

Legal — _____

Future — _____

Outsider — _____

Clause — _____

LUNCH (2ND FRIDAY)

Garden vegetable salad with chicken, and vinaigrette dressing
Iced tea or seltzer with lemon

AFTERNOON STRESS RELEASE (2ND FRIDAY)

Sit comfortably or lie down. If possible, do the following with your eyes closed: take a deep breath in, and then let it out slowly. Focus attention on your head and scalp, and imagine releasing all the tension there. Bring your focus down to your facial muscles and release that tension. Let the relaxed feeling extend through your cheeks and jaw, down into your neck and shoulders, releasing the tension there while breathing in and out slowly and deeply. Continue moving systematically down your body through your arms, hands, abdomen, back, hips, legs, and toes. Continue to breathe deeply for 1 to 3 minutes, allowing more tension to leave your body with each exhale.

AFTERNOON SNACK (2ND FRIDAY)

½ cup yogurt with 1 tablespoon raisins mixed in OR Peanut Butter/Ricotta
    Spread* on celery sticks
Plum or pear
Iced tea or water with lemon

AFTERNOON MENTAL AEROBICS (2ND FRIDAY)

Let's work on names and faces again. Tonight you will meet Fern Lambert. In
anticipation of this meeting, I want you to create a mental snapshot for her
name. To do this, visualize 3 SNAPs: one for her first name, another for the
first syllable of her last name, and a third for the second syllable of her last
name. Now, CONNECT the three SNAPs in your mind's eye.

DINNER (2ND FRIDAY)

Tomato, avocado, and sweet onion salad drizzled with olive oil and vinegar
Grilled 4 to 6 ounce salmon steak with herbs
Steamed Brussels sprouts
½ cup brown rice OR Wild Rice*
Frozen fruit or fruit juice bar OR Featherweight Cheesecake*
Seltzer, decaf iced tea, water, and/or a glass of wine

EVENING FITNESS/STRESS RELEASE (2ND FRIDAY)

10 to 15 minute after-dinner walk.

OR: repeat this morning's Wake-Up Stretch and Conditioning routine.

Drink a glass of water.

EVENING MENTAL AEROBICS (2ND FRIDAY)

Now we get to meet Fern Lambert. Focus on her face below and notice a distinguishing feature. *CONNECT* the earlier "name" *SNAP* to the "face" *SNAP*.

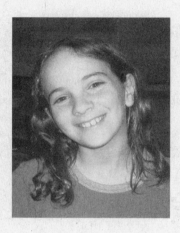

NIGHTTIME SNACK (2ND FRIDAY)

Banana

OR

Frozen banana/peanut-butter sandwich: ½ banana sliced lengthwise, spread 1 teaspoon peanut butter in middle, wrap in tin foil and freeze.

2ND SATURDAY (DAY THIRTEEN)

Tip for the Day: Many people complain of fatigue after lunch or during the afternoon. Sticking with the healthy brain diet—low in animal fats and smaller, more frequent meals and snacks—often cures this complaint. Others find additional stretching exercises, stress release/relaxation techniques, and aerobic conditioning breaks to be helpful remedies.

WAKE-UP STRETCH AND CONDITIONING (2ND SATURDAY)

Stretch #1 [*Deep Breathing Dips*]

Stretch # 2 [*Side Stretch*]

Stretch # 3 [*Chest/Back Expander*]

Conditioning Exercise # 1[*Russian Dancer Knee Lifts*] for a count of **50**.

Conditioning Exercise # 2 [*Marching Soldier*] for a count of **30**.

Conditioning Exercise # 3 [*Standing Crunches*] for a count of **30**.

Drink a glass of water.

BREAKFAST (2ND SATURDAY)

Open-face egg-white sandwich (2 cooked egg whites on 1 slice sourdough
toast with 1 ounce cheddar cheese and tomato or natural jam)
Fresh pineapple slices
Tea, coffee, water, or sparkling juice
Vitamin supplements

MORNING MENTAL AEROBICS (2ND SATURDAY)

I want you to meet two friends of mine, Bonnie and Sam. Use *LOOK, SNAP, CONNECT* to remember their names and faces.

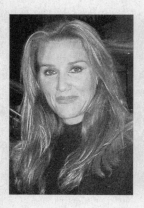 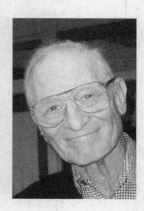

WEEKEND FITNESS (2ND SATURDAY)

15 to 30 minute morning walk.

OR: Treadmill, bicycle, workout of your choice.

Drink a glass of water.

MID-MORNING SNACK (2ND SATURDAY)

½ apple, sliced
½ cup low-fat cottage cheese OR Peanut Butter/Ricotta Spread*
Green tea or water

MID-MORNING MENTAL AEROBICS (2ND SATURDAY)

One more stab at the word pairs:

Necktie—Cellophane
Shadow—Net
Xylophone—Artichoke
Monkey—Raft
Moped—Icicle
Sedan—Banker

LUNCH (2ND SATURDAY)

Grilled turkey-dog on rye toast with sauerkraut and mustard
Orange sections
Iced tea or seltzer with lemon

AFTERNOON STRESS RELEASE (2ND SATURDAY)

Lie down or sit comfortably and breathe in slowly through your nose. Visualize your breath as it enters your sinuses, flows down into your chest, and expands your rib cage. Slowly breathe out through your nose, following the breath as it rises through your chest and sinuses, and finally leaves your body. Repeat slowly for 1 to 2 minutes.

AFTERNOON SNACK (2ND SATURDAY)

Sliced raw vegetables
String cheese OR Hummus Dip*
Iced tea or water with lemon

AFTERNOON MENTAL AEROBICS (2ND SATURDAY)

Show off your word-pair memorization expertise:

Necktie—_____
Shadow—_____

Xylophone — _____

Monkey — _____

Moped — _____

Sedan — _____

DINNER (2ND SATURDAY)

Arugula and shaved Parmesan cheese salad tossed in balsamic vinegar and
    olive oil dressing

Sliced 6-ounce chicken breast with fettuccine and tomato sauce

Steamed zucchini rounds

Sliced strawberries drizzled with 1 teaspoon chocolate sauce, and chopped
    peanuts

Seltzer, decaf iced tea, water, and/or a glass of wine

EVENING FITNESS/STRESS RELEASE (2ND SATURDAY)

10 to 15 minute after-dinner walk.

OR: repeat this morning's Wake-Up Stretch and Conditioning routine.

Drink a glass of water.

EVENING MENTAL AEROBICS (2ND SATURDAY)

Put *LOOK, SNAP, CONNECT* to work and remember the names of my friends I just introduced . . .

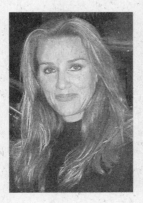 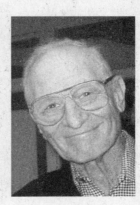

NIGHTTIME SNACK (2ND SATURDAY)

Popcorn (air-pop, hold the butter)

2ND SUNDAY (DAY FOURTEEN)

Tip for the Day: We can't memorize everything we see and hear because our brains, like computers, have limited short-term memory capacity. Most of us need to pick and choose what is most important to remember. Carrying a note-pad or pocket organizer allows us to keep a "memory list" of things to do, appointments to keep, etc., thus freeing our brain's storage space for learning and recall of fresh information such as new names and faces.

WAKE-UP STRETCH AND CONDITIONING (2ND SUNDAY)

Stretch #1 [*Deep Breathing Dips*]

Stretch #2 [*Side Stretch*]

Stretch #3 [*Chest/Back Expander*]

Conditioning Exercise #1 [*Russian Dancer Knee Lifts*] for a count of 50.

Conditioning Exercise #2 [*Marching Soldier*] for a count of 30.

Conditioning Exercise #3 [*Standing Crunches*] for a count of 30.

Drink a glass of water.

BREAKFAST (2ND SUNDAY)

Toasted onion bagel served with low-fat cream cheese, 1 slice smoked salmon, and tomato and onion as desired
Fresh or frozen mixed berries
Tea, coffee, water, or sparkling juice
Vitamin supplements

MORNING MENTAL AEROBICS (2ND SUNDAY)

Before leaving the house, think of four errands or tasks you need to accomplish today. Create a *SNAP* or visual image for each and then *CONNECT* them together in the order you plan to do them. Take your time and really let the images sink in.

WEEKEND FITNESS (2ND SUNDAY)

15 to 30 minute morning walk.

OR: Treadmill, bicycle, workout of your choice.

Drink a glass of water.

MID-MORNING SNACK (2ND SUNDAY)

Hard-boiled egg (or 3 egg whites)
1 cup vegetable soup of your choice
Green tea or water

MID-MORNING MENTAL AEROBICS (2ND SUNDAY)

Begin with your **one-minute stress release**.

Create SNAPs for each of the following names (see answers at the end of the section for suggestions if needed):

Ryan
Robertson
Shumann
Fabrikant
Carvette

LUNCH (2ND SUNDAY)

Salad Niçoise (butter lettuce with tuna, green beans, tomatoes, olives, egg whites, red pepper, and artichoke hearts, tossed in olive oil and vinegar dressing)
Iced tea or seltzer with lemon

AFTERNOON STRESS RELEASE (2ND SUNDAY)

Sit comfortably and imagine yourself at a beautiful beach just before sun-down. Breathe deeply and rhythmically as you conjure up the details of the setting. Feel the misty ocean breeze. Hear the seagulls and the waves. Watch as the sun touches the horizon and begins to slip below it, bit by bit—now half, three-quarters, almost gone, and finally completely disappeared. Take one more deep breath, close your eyes, and exhale slowly. Open your eyes before continuing with your day.

AFTERNOON SNACK (2ND SUNDAY)

Guacamole (mashed avocado, 2 tablespoons plain yogurt, ¼ cup drained
    salsa, and lemon juice to taste)
Sliced fresh vegetables OR Baked Corn Tortilla Chips*
Iced tea or water with lemon

AFTERNOON MENTAL AEROBICS (2ND SUNDAY)

Which three colors have been mixed up below?

UER   LREI   LLPA   PCD

DINNER (2ND SUNDAY)

Spinach salad with chopped apple and walnuts, and red wine vinegar and
    olive oil
Grilled 4 to 6 ounce sirloin steak (or chicken)
½ of a baked potato topped with chives OR corn-on-the-cob
Frozen yogurt OR Cinnamon Baked Apple*
Seltzer, decaf iced tea, water, and/or a glass of wine

EVENING FITNESS/STRESS RELEASE (2ND SUNDAY)

10 to 15 minute after-dinner walk.

OR: repeat this morning's Wake-Up Stretch and Conditioning routine.

Drink a glass of water.

EVENING MENTAL AEROBICS (2ND SUNDAY)

Did you remember to carry out your four errands from the morning?

Do you remember who this is?

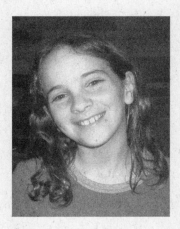

NIGHTTIME SNACK (2ND SUNDAY)

Fresh or frozen mixed berries

Answers to Mental Aerobics Exercises

1ST MONDAY EVENING

36; the sequence goes 2×2; 3×3; 4×4, etc.

1ST TUESDAY EVENING

(1) SIRAP (the only *city* spelled backward—all the others are *countries* spelled backward).

(2) John and Jim are standing back to back.

1ST WEDNESDAY MID-MORNING

People who live in glass houses shouldn't throw stones.

1ST THURSDAY AFTERNOON

There is not just one correct answer, but here are some examples:

Frank: frankfurter
Dinah: diner
Mike: microphone
Simon: Paul Simon
Barbara: barber
Jim: gymnasium
Phillip: Phillips screwdriver
George: gorge

1ST THURSDAY EVENING

To group the items, you need to recognize the categories: paperwork (facsimile, memo, Post-it, IOU), bodies of water (pond, lagoon, pool, lake), and jokes (pun, jibe, punch line, gag).

1ST SATURDAY MORNING

In order to group the items, you need to recognize the categories: edibles (pepper, cocoa, licorice, lentil), stringy objects (noose, dental floss, suture, wick), and containers (tobacco tin, drawer, shoebox, vial).

1ST SATURDAY EVENING

In the first box, the letter O is the only vowel (it is also the only letter without a line in it). In the second box, the number 35 is the only one that cannot be divided by 2 or 3.

1ST SUNDAY MID-MORNING

Here are some possible approaches:
Maremont: a *mare* running up a *mount*ain
Laghrissi: a *log* with *grease*
Marseille: a *sail* boat on the planet *Mars*

2ND MONDAY AFTERNOON

Paul: pole
Foreman: a foreman on the job or four men
Create a story: four men lifting a pole

2ND MONDAY EVENING

Paul Foreman has a high forehead. See four men lifting a pole on his forehead.

2ND WEDNESDAY AFTERNOON

P	O	R	T
O	V	E	R
R	E	D	O
T	R	O	T

2ND WEDNESDAY EVENING

The only piece with more sides on the inner shape than the outer one:

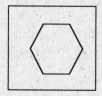

2ND WEDNESDAY EVENING

Here are some suggestions:

Social: a group of people chatting
Pressure: tire gauge
Outstanding: one person's head standing out above a crowd
Hate: an angry face

2ND SUNDAY MID-MORNING

Here are some possible approaches:

Ryan: rye bread
Robertson: Julia Roberts with a son
Shumann: a man selling shoes

Fabrikant: fabric in a cantor's hand
Carvette: the famous sports car (Corvette)

2ND SUNDAY AFTERNOON

PURPLE, RED, LILAC

Optional Food Substitutions

You may substitute any day's breakfast menu with 3 egg whites scrambled plus 1 toast and fresh fruit, or 1 cup of cold raisin-bran cereal with ½ cup non-fat milk and berries. Frozen berries have as much of an antioxidant punch as fresh ones, but be sure to use the naturally frozen variety and avoid fruit in sugary syrups. All mid-morning and afternoon snack selections may be replaced by a choice of the following:

1. A snack-bag of cut raw vegetables (bell pepper, carrots, tomatoes, etc.) plus 1 ounce string cheese;

2. 1 cup chicken or vegetable bouillon or soup, plus a hard boiled egg (or 3 egg whites) or 1 ounce string cheese;

3. A fruit and yogurt smoothie (consider neighborhood juice shops) or 1 cup plain yogurt mixed with fresh or frozen strawberries and ½ banana.

Lunch menus may be substituted by a vegetable salad containing approximately 4 ounces of chicken or tuna, plus 2 whole grain crackers, and fresh fruit or a fruit sorbet.

Dinner menus may be replaced by a grilled 4 to 6 ounce fish fillet or chicken breast, steamed vegetable, ½ cup brown rice, and berries or yogurt for dessert. For people who do not like or cannot tolerate cheese, they can get their necessary calcium from supplements or other food sources such as kale, green vegetables, or alternate milk products. You may substitute lean meats, tofu, or eggs for other sources of protein.

Nighttime snacks are optional—fresh fruit or frozen fruit-juice bars are good substitutions for the indicated choice.

Chapter Four:

Your 2-Week Checkup—
Gauge Your Success

I have a memory like an elephant. In fact, elephants often consult me.
— NOËL COWARD

Now that you have completed the 14-Day Memory Prescription, this chapter will give you an opportunity to reassess your objective and subjective memory abilities, your daily stress levels, and your physical conditioning status. By comparing these "after" assessment results with your "before" baseline scores, you will be able to gauge your improvement from your first two weeks on the plan. In addition, you can gain valuable information with which to further tailor your Memory Prescription to meet your individual needs. This two-week checkup will help you decide if there are any areas of the program you'd like to make adjustments to as you renew your prescription. Upcoming chapters provide many modification options.

After their initial two weeks, most of my patients and UCLA study volunteers report improved memory scores, lower stress levels, greater physical stamina, and for some, measurable weight loss. Many stated that their friends and family members made comments about how much better they *looked*.

Another benefit of completing the assessment tools once again and witnessing your improvement is the feeling of empowerment it brings. This sense that you can improve your memory abilities will fuel your confidence, and our research shows that this confidence alone leads to further memory improvements.

After each of the assessments, add up your score and record it in the space provided. Then turn to page 31 to compare your earlier scores to the new ones.

Update Your Objective Memory Assessment Score

The 14-Day Plan provided daily opportunities to develop your basic memory skills and learn some more advanced memory techniques. Let's see how much better you are at learning and recalling a new list of 10 words. The following list includes words different from the first word list but of similar difficulty level for committing to memory and recalling after a 20-minute break.

Because the assessment is timed, you will again need a stopwatch, kitchen timer, or timepiece with a second hand before beginning. The test involves learning a new list of 10 words over a 2-minute period and recalling them after a 20-minute break. When ready, set your timer for two minutes, then read and learn the words on the list in Objective Memory Assessment No. 2.

OBJECTIVE MEMORY ASSESSMENT NO. 2
STUDY THE FOLLOWING WORDS
FOR UP TO TWO MINUTES:

Salad
Butterfly
Nun
Locker
Ankle
Truck
Candy

Sunset

Rattle

Tile

When your two minutes are up, put aside *The Memory Prescription*, reset your timer for a 20-minute break, and do something else—return some phone calls, weed the lawn, whatever you like, just make sure you distract yourself from the word list with something else. After 20 minutes, write down as many of the words as you can recall and record the total number below.

Objective Memory Total Score, Day 14:_____

Fill in that number in the chart on page 31. Most people who follow *The Memory Prescription* plan show improvement in their score. For people with relatively high scores at baseline (8 or 9), the room for improvement on this test is minimal. This does not mean that your memory has not improved. It simply means that the test was not challenging enough for you to show improvement. You are still likely to show subjective memory improvement on the next questionnaire.

Assessing Your Subjective Memory Ability

Now let's see how you rate your own subjective memory abilities after completing the 14-Day Plan. On the next pages you'll find another memory self-awareness questionnaire. Answer the following questions by circling the number between 1 and 7 that best reflects how you judge your own memory ability.

SUBJECTIVE MEMORY QUESTIONNAIRE

How would you rate your overall memory?	Poor		Good			Excellent	
	1	2	3	4	5	6	7

How often do these present a problem for you?	Always		Sometimes			Never	
names	1	2	3	4	5	6	7
faces	1	2	3	4	5	6	7
appointments	1	2	3	4	5	6	7
where I put things (e.g., keys, eyeglasses)	1	2	3	4	5	6	7
performing household chores	1	2	3	4	5	6	7
directions to places	1	2	3	4	5	6	7
phone numbers I have just checked	1	2	3	4	5	6	7
phone numbers I use frequently	1	2	3	4	5	6	7
things people tell me	1	2	3	4	5	6	7
keeping up correspondence	1	2	3	4	5	6	7
personal dates (e.g., birthdays)	1	2	3	4	5	6	7
words	1	2	3	4	5	6	7
forgetting what I wanted to buy at the store	1	2	3	4	5	6	7
taking a test	1	2	3	4	5	6	7
beginning something and forgetting what I was doing	1	2	3	4	5	6	7
losing my thread of thought in conversation	1	2	3	4	5	6	7
losing my thread of thought in public speaking	1	2	3	4	5	6	7

knowing whether I have already told
someone something

1 2   3 4 5   6 7

**As you read a novel, how often do you have
trouble remembering what you have read . . .**

	Always	Sometimes	Never

in opening chapters, once I've finished
the book?

1 2   3 4 5   6 7

3 or 4 chapters before the one I'm now reading?   1 2   3 4 5   6 7

in the chapter before the one I'm now reading?   1 2   3 4 5   6 7

in the paragraph just before the one
I'm now reading?

1 2   3 4 5   6 7

in the sentence just before the one I'm
now reading?

1 2   3 4 5   6 7

How well do you remember things that occurred . . .

	Poorly	Fair	Well

last month?

1 2   3 4 5   6 7

between six months and one year ago?

1 2   3 4 5   6 7

between one and five years ago?

1 2   3 4 5   6 7

between six and ten years ago?

1 2   3 4 5   6 7

**When you read a newspaper or magazine article,
how often do you have trouble remembering
what you have read . . .**

	Always	Sometimes	Never

in the opening paragraphs, once I have
finished the article?

1 2   3 4 5   6 7

3 or 4 paragraphs before the one I am
currently reading?

1 2   3 4 5   6 7

in the paragraph before the one I am
currently reading?

1 2   3 4 5   6 7

3 or 4 sentences before the one I am
currently reading?   1   2   3   4   5   6   7

in the sentence before the one I am
currently reading?   1   2   3   4   5   6   7

Add up all the numbers you have circled and write in your sum below.

Subjective Memory Total Score, Day 14: _____

Compare this score to your previous score on page 31. Note how much better you feel about your current memory abilities compared to two weeks ago. You may feel inspired by your reassessment scores to further refine the memory training component of your Memory Prescription to meet your personal needs. The modification chapters can show you how to increase or decrease the level of difficulty of the exercises, as well as introduce new games and puzzles.

Reassess Your Stress Level

During the past two weeks, you have spent time each day practicing stress release exercises. If you had done only these exercises and no other part of the 14-Day Plan, you would most likely be experiencing reduced daily stress. However, you have had the added benefit of regular physical aerobic conditioning and a healthy brain diet to contribute to your overall sense of well-being. Retake the stress level questionnaire, record your total score below, and then transfer the score to the chart on page 32 to compare your current rating to your baseline.

STRESS LEVEL QUESTIONNAIRE

How would you rate your overall stress level?	Low		Medium			High	
	1	2	3	4	5	6	7

To what degree do the following situations make you tense or irritable?	Little		Somewhat			Very	
argument with friend or relative	1	2	3	4	5	6	7
waiting for a table in a restaurant	1	2	3	4	5	6	7
arriving late for an appointment	1	2	3	4	5	6	7
forgetting someone's name	1	2	3	4	5	6	7
anticipating work deadlines	1	2	3	4	5	6	7
last minute changes in plans	1	2	3	4	5	6	7

How easy is it for you to relax when you . . .	Easy		Medium			Difficult	
watch a television show or movie?	1	2	3	4	5	6	7
read a book or magazine?	1	2	3	4	5	6	7
take a walk, jog, or do other physical exercise?	1	2	3	4	5	6	7

How often do you experience each of the following?	Never		Sometimes			Always	
insomnia	1	2	3	4	5	6	7
shortness of breath	1	2	3	4	5	6	7
rapid heart rate	1	2	3	4	5	6	7
cold hands or feet	1	2	3	4	5	6	7
impatience	1	2	3	4	5	6	7
irritability	1	2	3	4	5	6	7

indecisiveness	1	2		3	4	5		6	7
tension or worry	1	2		3	4	5		6	7

Stress Level Total Score, Day 14: _____

Reassess Your Level of Physical Fitness

The 14-Day Plan gave you a chance to improve your aerobic conditioning and stamina with modest but steady increases in your training level. To reassess your physical fitness level after the first two weeks of the plan, complete the following questionnaire by circling the number from 1 to 7 for each question that best describes your current physical fitness level.

PHYSICAL FITNESS QUESTIONNAIRE

To what degree might the following activities make you feel short of breath?

	Minimal		Somewhat			Very	
playing table tennis for 10 minutes	1	2	3	4	5	6	7
walking briskly for 10 minutes	1	2	3	4	5	6	7
jogging for 10 minutes	1	2	3	4	5	6	7
climbing a flight of stairs	1	2	3	4	5	6	7
climbing three flights of stairs	1	2	3	4	5	6	7

How sore would you be after each of the following activities?

	Minimal		Somewhat			Very	
sweeping floors for 10 minutes	1	2	3	4	5	6	7
carrying grocery bags for 10 minutes	1	2	3	4	5	6	7

carrying a 20-pound suitcase for 10 minutes	1	2	3	4	5	6	7
riding a bicycle for 30 minutes	1	2	3	4	5	6	7
playing two sets of tennis	1	2	3	4	5	6	7

Add up your total score, which can range from 10 to 70, and record it below, then turn to page 32 to see how much more fit you feel today compared to when you began the Plan.

Physical Fitness Total Score, Day 14: _____

Weighing in on Day 14

Many people are diet fanatics—they obsess over every calorie or half-gram of fat, they weigh meal portions religiously, and they jump on their bathroom scale a half-dozen times each day. The Memory Prescription Diet was designed to maximize brain health and fitness; however, weight loss has become a secondary benefit for many people—even in the first two weeks of their program—without much effort. Weigh yourself today and compare this number with the amount you weighed two weeks ago (page 32). See if your weight has remained stable or if you may have lost any pounds during the first two weeks of your Memory Prescription. In Chapter 7, I offer advice on how to adjust the diet component of your prescription to increase or decrease your weight while working toward quality longevity.

14-Day Body Weight: _____

Primed and Ready

You have now completed your 14-Day Memory Prescription plan, and you are probably feeling pretty good physically and mentally. Chances are friends and family members may be commenting on your radiance and energy level.

I have found that something else happens to a person at the end of these first two weeks—they get hooked on the Memory Prescription habit. They now crave the energy, mental acuity, and sense of well-being they attained from the plan and they don't want to give it up. This was my hope from the outset: to get you primed for a Memory Prescription renewal.

Several of the following chapters contain updates on some of the latest scientific findings that support each of the components of the plan, particularly the Big 4: stress reduction, mental aerobics and memory training, the Memory Prescription Diet, and physical aerobic conditioning. You'll also find out about the latest medicines, hormones, vitamins, and supplements that may or may not protect or boost your brainpower. Chapter 11 contains worksheets and specific strategies that will help you fine-tune your Memory Prescription renewal and tailor it to fit into your lifestyle needs.

Chapter Five:

Pump Up Your Mental Aerobics

I sometimes worry about my short attention span, but not for very long.
— HERB CAEN

I love doing crossword puzzles. Every morning I rush outside to get my daily *Times*—L.A. and New York—anticipating those puzzles. As I read through the local and national news, the business, lifestyle and theater sections, I look forward to those puzzles—saving them for the very end, like some great reward or delicious, tempting dessert. What? You don't do that?

Most newspaper crossword fans know that the difficulty level of a particular puzzle is distinctly related to the day of the week—as we get closer to the weekend, the puzzles steadily become more challenging. Not long ago I found a helpful book for boosting my crossword confidence: *The New York Times Daily Crossword Puzzles: Monday.* I felt nearly brilliant when working those puzzles and wouldn't fret if my last pencil lead broke because I could do those Monday puzzles in ink—no need for an eraser here, thank you. Those puzzles were just the right level of difficulty for me, just challenging enough to be fun and interesting; not too easy or boring, yet not too difficult or frustrating.

You too will get the most out of your mental aerobic exercises when you choose activities that are the right level for you. Crossword puzzles are a good example of *mental aerobics*, tasks or exercises that involve mental effort. The goal of these exercises is to "shake up" our usual mental assumptions and force us to think of novel solutions. A successful brainteaser or puzzle often gives us a moment of pleasure and satisfaction when we stumble upon the solution—at that moment a "lightbulb" of understanding and insight turns on in our brain. Some experts believe this process correlates with the actual "stretching and toning" workout we are aiming to achieve for our brain cells.

The 14-Day Memory Prescription emphasizes mental aerobics that specifically improve memory performance, but just as I enjoy my "crossword fix," many people may wish to benefit from additional stimulation of the brain's memory cells. This chapter includes more brainteasers and puzzles for augmenting your Memory Prescription mental aerobics routine and provides an update on the latest research that has convinced many to train their brains as a strategy to stave off future memory loss.

High-Impact Mental Aerobics

Several large studies have found a lower risk for developing Alzheimer's disease in intellectually active people compared with their mentally stagnant counterparts. And the mental activity can take many forms, such as reading, working jigsaw puzzles, woodworking, painting, knitting, and playing board games. Some studies have even found that people with mentally demanding jobs—professionals, managers, etc.—experience less memory decline as they age when compared with their counterparts who have less demanding jobs.

Dr. Joe Verghese and his associates at the Albert Einstein College of Medicine in New York asked 469 older adults how often they participated in leisure activities like dancing, playing cards, or doing crossword puzzles. Over the years, the scientists kept track of who developed mild memory loss or full-blown dementia. They found that the people who were the most active mentally had a 63 percent lower risk of getting dementia compared with those who rarely played board games, read, or did similar activities. The people who played the most had the most protection: doing crossword puzzles four days each week translated into a 47 percent lower risk of dementia compared with once-a-week puzzle solvers. For each day of the week that people exercised their minds, the researchers found nearly a 10 percent reduction in the risk for dementia.

Other studies indicate that mental activity earlier in life is protective as well. Scientists at Case Western Reserve University in Cleveland, Ohio, found that the rate for developing Alzheimer's disease was three times lower in people who had been intellectually active during their forties and fifties compared with those who had not. Rush University researchers have found that mental activity as early as one's twenties predicted better cognitive function late in life. This work is consistent with many other studies showing that college graduates have a lower risk for developing Alzheimer's disease than those who never get beyond a high school education.

Experts believe that one reason solving puzzles and other forms of mental stimulation help lower the risk for dementia is that people develop a "cognitive reserve" that allows them to tolerate more damage from Alzheimer's and other brain diseases. A recent study by Dr. Yaakov Stern and colleagues at Columbia University in New York suggests that it's not how much brain you have, but how you use it that makes the difference. The investigators tested 19 people with a range of IQs from below to above average. Participants performed memory tasks while the investigators measured their brain activity patterns during functional MRI scans.

The scans showed more activity in the frontal lobes of people with higher intelligence. These same investigators also have demonstrated the brain-protective effects of education. These findings show that more intelligent and better educated people use their brains differently than those without these benefits, and this may help explain why keeping the mind active helps protect against the onset of Alzheimer's disease.

Mental aerobics may not only keep our brain cells healthy, but they may also help them grow. New research suggests that the brain can actually rewire itself and grow new cells, a process known as *neurogenesis*, believed impossible until the last few decades. Dr. Elizabeth Gould of Princeton University has shown that, well into adult life, laboratory animals continue to produce new brain cells in the hippocampus, that sea horse shaped formation beneath the temples. Dr. Fred Gage and his associates at the Salk Institute have shown that such neurogenesis can occur in humans as well. Using a chemical marker that shows dividing cells, he found that patients who had died from cancer had evidence of such cell division. Given the stress of fighting a disease like cancer and how such stress inhibits neurogenesis, we might expect to see even greater degrees of neurogenesis in a healthy individual.

Drs. Gage and William Greenough of the University of Illinois have helped us understand that neurogenesis may be an important aspect of memory and learning. In their animal studies, they have found that enriched environments are associated with greater numbers of synapses or cell communication links in the brain's memory centers. And, when running through their mazes and completing other memory tests, the stimulated animals appear more intelligent. These kinds of studies have led many researchers to believe that routine mental exercise stimulates existing connections between neurons and leads to new neuronal connections in the brain.

Even in the face of this and other compelling evidence for the protective benefits of mental aerobics, there are still skeptics who believe that mental activity has little or no effect on the rate at which our brains age. However, even without absolute proof of cause and effect, the risks of staying mentally active are minimal, and the potential gains great. In other words, remaining mentally active and practicing mental aerobic exercises can't hurt. It can also enrich our lives considerably.

Studies on mental aerobics have shown that the tasks must involve an element of effort. They can be diverse and can include any of a number of activities: reading, working jigsaw puzzles, woodworking, painting, knitting, or playing board games. You may prefer learning a language or reading a challenging novel or biography. Evidence indicates that the "fun factor" keeps us coming back for more, and that is what you want—to sustain the activity over time. Epidemiological studies suggest that we need to develop a regular habit of mental aerobics, and that years of activity may be needed to obtain optimum effect.

Cross Train Your Brain

If you work out with a physical fitness trainer, they will have you focus on working one group of muscles one day, and a different group of muscles the next. In this way, you are less likely to injure yourself and you are more able to balance your strength and stamina.

I like to apply the same principle to mental aerobic workouts by sorting the exercises according to which brain hemisphere we're toning. For most people, left-brain functions include logical analysis (reasoning, drawing conclusions), information sequencing (making lists, organizing thoughts), language and speech, reading and writing, counting and mathematics, and symbol recognition. The right hemisphere gets involved in spatial tasks such as reading maps, staying oriented, and finding our way, as well as in artistic and musical abilities, face recognition, depth perception, dreaming, emotional perception, and sense of humor. In left-handed people, these hemispheric functions are reversed.

Ideally, you want to work both hemispheres, and you may want to alternate your mental aerobic stimulation program from left hemisphere to right hemisphere. A recent study showed how a specific form of right brain activity like reading maps can affect the size of the hippocampus, a key brain region involved in spatial memory.

In this investigation, London taxi drivers spent two years studying for a difficult exam about the city streets. When the taxi drivers were asked to imagine a specific route in the city, a brain scan imaging study showed that the hippocampus was working. These same scientists have recently reported that the size of the hippocampus in these taxi drivers is larger than average and that its size varies directly with the number of years on the job. Other studies have found that it need not take two years to demonstrate training benefits. For example, University of Rochester researchers found that playing video games for only 10 days can result in improved right-brain performance scores. Our goal in mental aerobics is to build both sides of the brain and alternate such right-brain exercises as mazes and map reading with left-brain verbal and logic tasks.

Aerobicize Your Mind

The 14-Day Memory Prescription includes mental aerobic exercises as warm-ups to help you develop practical everyday memory techniques (Chapter 6). Some readers may wish to augment their mental aerobic workout during the first two weeks of their program. In addition, I recommend that everyone create some kind of mental aerobics routine to help build brain efficiency over time, particularly beyond the initial two-week program. Keep in mind the following guidelines when individualizing your mental aerobic workout:

- Like any exercise routine, the more fun you have, the easier it will be for you to maintain your program over the long haul. Choose activities that you enjoy, whether it's playing a musical instrument or computer games, reading mystery novels or classics, or perhaps solving brainteasers and puzzles. No one form of exercise has been shown to be more effective than another, so look to your own personal preferences as a guide to individualizing your program.

- Build brainpower by starting with simple exercises and moving up to more complex ones. In this way, you can continue to flex and tone your "brain muscles" while developing mental stamina and efficiency. Mental stimulation exercises should be challenging, but pace yourself and have reasonable expectations.

- People with mentally taxing jobs may wish to play down or even avoid a daily mental aerobic workout. The stress reduction component may need more emphasis to balance such mentally taxing lifestyles.

- Work both sides of your brain and alternate your mental aerobic stimulation program from left hemisphere to right hemisphere exercises.

The following exercises are divided according to beginning, intermediate, and advanced levels, as well as which part of the brain each exercise trains. Before trying them, take a moment to review the results of your subjective and objective memory scores (Chapter 2 if you have not yet done your 14-Day Plan, Chapter 4 if you have). These will point you to your optimal level to begin or continue your program.

When performing the exercises, notice how they make you feel. If you feel yourself getting frustrated quickly, go back and start at a less advanced level. If you find the exercises too easy, move on to the more advanced. Once you know the kind of mental aerobics that works best for you, you may want to expand your repertoire by seeking additional resources at the library or on the Internet. The key is to determine the right exercise level for you and build up gradually from that point. Be creative—look outside the realm of normal thinking, and have fun.

BEGINNING EXERCISES

1. **Warm-up Exercise.** Try using your non-dominant hand (i.e., left hand if you are right-handed) in a routine task like brushing your teeth or hair. (I urge you to avoid trying the non-dominant hand exercise during your morning shave until you are at the very advanced stage or you have lots of Band-Aids handy.)

2. **Right-Brain Exercise.** How many triangles can you find in the following figure?

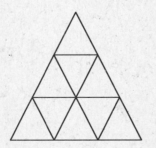

3. *Right-Brain Excercise.* Complete the sequence by choosing object A, B, or C:

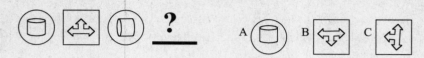

4. *Right-Brain Exercise.* Look at the object on the left and then choose the version that matches: A, B, C, or D.

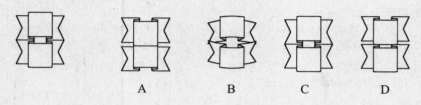

A   B   C   D

5. *Right-Brain Exercise.* Which of the three numbered pieces below will complete the sequence?

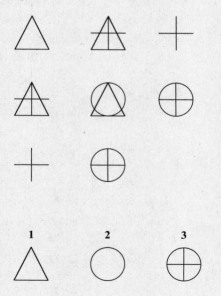

1   2   3

6. Left-Brain Exercise. Unscramble the letters to find the two words that name an Academy Award–winning buddy movie from the 1970s.

GHTIENTS

7. Left-Brain Exercise. Make three words from the following jumbled letters.

REHTEDOSWR

8. Left-Brain Exercise. Jim is twice as old as his brother Jeff. Ten years later, however, Jeff has caught up and is now two-thirds his brother's age. How can that be?

9. Left-Brain Exercise. What five-letter word becomes smaller when you add two letters to it? Clue: Who wrote this zany question?

10. Left-Brain Exercise. You have two coins for a total of 35 cents and you know that one is *not* a dime. What are the two coins?

11. Left-Brain Exercise. Fill in the missing letter and number below:

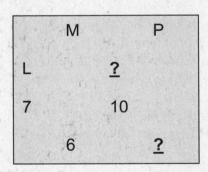

12. **Whole-Brain Exercise (both hemispheres).** Figure out the word suggested by the message in the box.

```
┌─────────────────────────────────┐
│                                 │
│            CYCLE                │
│            CYCLE                │
│            CYCLE                │
│                                 │
└─────────────────────────────────┘
```

13. **Whole-Brain Exercise.** You toss a quarter and you have the re-markable luck of it landing heads 20 times in a row. What are the odds that it will be heads on the next toss?

ANSWERS TO BEGINNING EXERCISES

1. **Warm-up Exercise.** No right answer.

2. **Right-Brain Exercise.** The total number of triangles is 13 (don't forget the combinations of triangles within triangles).

3. **Right-Brain Exercise.** C.

4. **Right-Brain Exercise.** C.

5. **Right-Brain Exercise.** 2 (The last symbol in each column and row is always the same as the preceding two symbols minus any part that has been duplicated.)

6. **Left-Brain Exercise.** "The Sting"

7. **Left-Brain Exercise.** Two correct answers: either THREE WORDS or THE RED ROWS.

8. **Left-Brain Exercise.** When Jim was 20 years old and Jeff was 10, Jim was twice his brother's age. Ten years later, Jim reached his thirtieth birthday and Jeff his twentieth, so Jeff was two-thirds his brother's age (20 over 30 = ⅔).

9. **Left-Brain Exercise.** "Small" gets "smaller" when you add two letters.

10. **_Left-Brain Exercise._** A quarter and a dime (one is not a dime but the other is).

11. **_Left-Brain Exercise._** The letter "O" completes the alphabetical sequence and the number "9" completes the numerical sequence.

12. **_Whole-Brain Exercise._** Tricycle.

13. **_Whole-Brain Exercise._** The odds will be 50:50 for heads on the next toss. This would be the case even if you flipped heads 100 times or a 1,000 times in a row.

The above beginning exercises may have taxed your brain a bit, so before moving on, try a stress reduction exercise, maybe a two-minute deep breathing break or a stretching routine. If you found these exercises at the right level of challenge for you now, then consider checking out the latest Web sites and other resources for puzzles and brainteasers with similar levels of difficulty.

Once you're comfortable at this level, then try advancing to the next group of exercises for a tougher brain workout.

INTERMEDIATE EXERCISES

1. **_Warm-up Exercise._** Challenge your brain's usual way of doing things by taking a newspaper, book, or magazine and reading it upside down. Since you are not used to this way of reading, the letters will look like gibberish at first. If you take your time, you will begin to make sense of it, and with practice, you will build your upside down reading abilities. This is a great exercise for any would-be yoga masters who might like to catch up on reading while standing on their heads.

2. *Right-Brain Exercise.* See if you can reverse the direction of this triangle by only moving three of the smiling faces.

3. *Right-Brain Exercise.* Create a "virtual triangle" by rearranging these three Pac-Man icons.

4. *Right-Brain Exercise.* Mazes are great ways to train your visual-spatial skills. See how you do on this one.

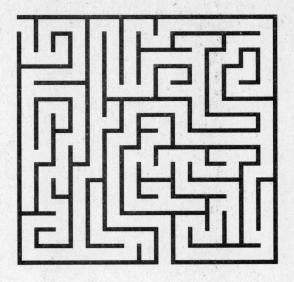

5. **Right-Brain Exercise.** Figure out which tile completes the sequence:

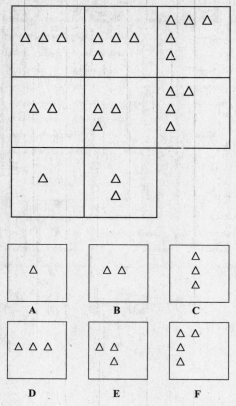

6. **Left-Brain Exercise.** Unscramble the letters to find another Academy Award–winning film.

ENECLARW FO BIRAAA

7. **Left-Brain Exercise.** Which is the odd one out?

DACHSHUND POODLE SHEPHERD BEAGLE

8. *Left-Brain Exercise.* Assume that none of the following statements is true and try to figure out who spilled the red wine on the white carpet.

Gary: Diane spilled the wine.
Dick: Gary will tell you who spilled the wine.
Angie: Dick, Gary, and I could not have spilled the wine.
Steve: I did not spill the wine.
Andy: Gary spilled the wine, so Dick and Angie could not have done it.
Dean: I spilled the wine, so Dick is innocent.

9. *Left-Brain Exercise.* An eight-letter word is hidden in the box below. You can find it by starting with the correct letter and moving counterclockwise or clockwise around the box's inner rim using each letter only once.

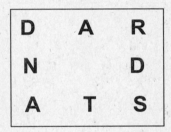

10. *Left-Brain Exercise.* A spider is trying to climb a 10-foot wall. Each hour, the spider climbs 5 feet up, but slides back 4 feet. How many hours does it take the spider to reach the top of the wall?

11. *Left-Brain Exercise.* Starting with the word SELL, change one letter at a time until you have the word FAIR. Each change must spell a proper word.

SELL

. . . .

. . . .

. . . .

FAIR

12. *Left-Brain Exercise.* Figure out the two ways that one of the following groups of letters differs from the others.

DNALGNE KRAMNED LAGUTROP NEDEWS MADERTSMA

13. *Whole-Brain Exercise.* Only one word in this paragraph is misspelled; see if you can spot it. You may have trouble concentrating enough to identify it initially, but I am confident that if you are vigilant, you will arrive at the answer.

14. *Whole-Brain Exercise.* Figure out the common phrase suggested by the message in the box.

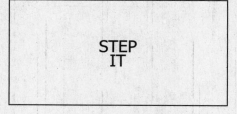

ANSWERS TO INTERMEDIATE EXERCISES

1. *Warm-up Exercise.* No right answer.

2. *Right-Brain Exercise.*

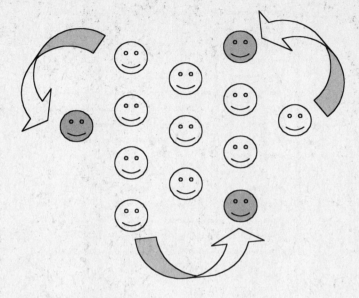

3. *Right-Brain Exercise.*

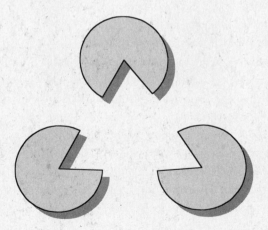

4. **Left-Brain Exercise.** The dotted line shows you the solution.

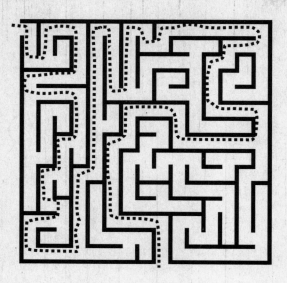

5. **Right-Brain Exercise.** C.

6. **Left-Brain Exercise.** "Lawrence of Arabia"

7. **Left-Brain Exercise.** Shepherd is the only word that has a common meaning beyond a dog breed.

8. **Left-Brain Exercise.** Steve should not be allowed to drink red wine on a white carpet because he spilled the wine. If the statement "I did not spill the wine" is definitely false, we can be certain that Steve spilled the wine. Statements that some people "could not have" spilled the wine only mean that these people could have spilled the wine, but do not guarantee that they did. Dean's statement that "Dick is innocent" is too vague. We know that Dick is not innocent, but this does not assure us that he spilled the wine.

9. **Left-Brain Exercise.** STANDARD.

10. **Left-Brain Exercise.** You might have answered 10 hours, but it only took the spider 6 hours to reach the top of the wall. The first hour, the spider climbs a height of 5 feet and then slides back 4 feet and thus ends up at a height of 1 foot. After the second hour, he reaches 6 feet and slides back to

2 feet. After the third hour, he reaches 7 feet but slides back to 3 feet. After the fourth hour, he reaches 8 feet but slides back to 4 feet. The fifth hour, he reaches nine feet, but slides back to 5 feet. At the end of the sixth hour, he reaches 10 feet, so he is *now* at the top of the wall.

11. ***Left-Brain Exercise.*** SELL, FELL, FALL, FAIL, FAIR

12. ***Left-Brain Exercise.*** All are European countries spelled backward except for "MADERTSMA," which is a European city misspelled backward.

13. ***Whole-Brain Exercise.*** The misspelled word is "mispelled."

14. ***Whole-Brain Exercise.*** Step on it.

Take a deep breath, perhaps a brisk power walk around the block, and snack on some omega-3/antioxidant brain food—perhaps a broccoli salad seasoned with olive oil, vinegar, and lemon juice with a side of smoked salmon. Now brace yourself for the high-impact mental aerobics that follow.

ADVANCED EXERCISES

1. ***Warm-up Exercise.*** You'll need a pencil and piece of paper for this handwriting warm-up. Try writing your name using your non-dominant hand (e.g., left hand if you are right-handed). After practicing a bit, give your left hand a break and write your name with your right hand, but do it so the letters come out upside down and backward. It may help if you write your name down the usual way so you have a right-side-up version to copy.

2. *Right-Brain Exercise*. Figure out which tile completes the sequence:

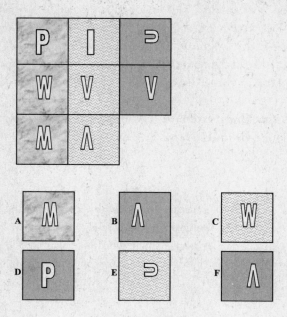

3. *Right-Brain Exercise*. Rearrange the three drawings below to create the letter "e." You can rotate them but do not change the angles or the lengths of the lines.

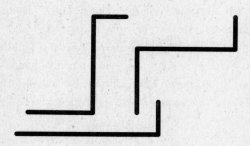

4. Right-Brain Exercise. You'll find the following maze a bit more challenging than the previous one.

5. Left-Brain Exercise. Most of us have squirmed through a white lie or a half-truth at some point. Can you identify the fibber in the puzzle below?

Robert says Bill lies, while Bill accuses Steve of lying. Steve claims that both Robert and Bill are liars.

6. Left-Brain Exercise. Can you unscramble the letters below to find three fruits?

D A E O A T P M O V A O C A T H O C

7. Left-Brain Exercise. Starting with the word MEATY, change one letter at a time until you have the word WALLS. Each change must spell a proper word.

MEATY

. . . .

. . . . .

. . . .

. . . .

WALLS

8. *Left-Brain Exercise.* Here's another Academy Award–winner, but with six words in its title.

EBETHDIRG NOHET VERRIWAIK

9. *Left-Brain Exercise.* Five men got out of two cars when it started to rain. They had no umbrellas, so four of them picked up their pace to stay dry while the fifth did not. However, it was the fifth man who remained dry while the others got soaked. How might you explain this?

10. *Left-Brain Exercise.* I want you to try and pick out what is unusual about this paragraph. How quickly you find out what is so unusual about it is an indication of your ability to think fast and to think in a way that shows off your smarts. I know that at first this paragraph looks ordinary, and you probably think that nothing is wrong with it. In fact, nothing is wrong with it, but it is unusual. Just study it long and hard, and you will know that which you first cannot hit upon. Think about it, and do it without any coaching. I know that your brain can find a way to get it right, so work hard to try to figure it out and stay cool throughout this task. Good luck.

11. *Whole-Brain Exercise.* Figure out the common phrase suggested by the message in the box.

HEA   DAC HE

12. Whole-Brain Exercise. A fisherman is on his favorite bridge trying to catch some Atlantic salmon swimming upstream to spawn. He notices a particularly large one swimming at a steady pace. After a mile, the salmon passes a morsel of rainbow smelt floating downstream. The salmon continues swimming upstream for half an hour and then turns around and swims back to catch up to the smelt for a snack. The salmon and the smelt arrive at the bridge at the same time, and the salmon has kept swimming at the same speed. Can you figure out the speed of the river?

ANSWERS TO ADVANCED EXERCISES

1. **Warm-up Exercise.** No right answer.
2. **Right-Brain Exercise.** F.
3. **Right-Brain Exercise.**

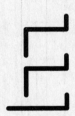

4. *Right-Brain Exercise.*

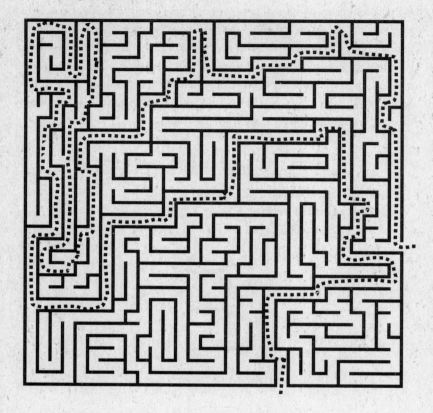

5. *Left-Brain Exercise.* If Robert is lying, then Bill is telling the truth. If Robert is telling the truth, then Bill is lying. Robert and Bill can't both be telling the truth or both lying; therefore, Steve must be lying.

If Robert is telling the truth, then Bill's lie means that Steve is telling the truth. But we've already established Steve as a liar, so Robert also can't be telling the truth.

If Bill is telling the truth, then Robert must have lied. That also means that Steve is lying, which is certainly possible because he said that both

Robert and Bill were lying, and that is a lie about Bill. The only solution is that Bill is the only one among the three who is telling the truth.

    6. *Left-Brain Exercise*. PEACH, TOMATO, AVOCADO. Though we tend to think of tomatoes and avocados as vegetables since we mix them in our salads, their seeds get them into the fruit category.

    7. *Left-Brain Exercise*. MEATY, MEATS, MELTS, MALTS, MALLS, WALLS.

    8. *Left-Brain Exercise*. "The Bridge on the River Kwai."

    9. *Left-Brain Exercise*. The four men who picked up their pace were carrying the fifth man in a coffin.

    10. *Left-Brain Exercise*. The paragraph does not include the letter "e."

    11. *Whole-Brain Exercise*. Splitting headache.

    12. *Whole-Brain Exercise*. You don't need pages of mathematical formulas to solve this puzzle—just some simple deductive reasoning. Since the smelt is floating downstream, it has the same speed as the water. Thus, if the salmon is swimming upstream, away from the smelt for half an hour, it will take him another half hour to swim back to the smelt. Because the salmon is swimming with constant speed relative to the speed of the water, it helps to think as though the river water doesn't move, so the smelt doesn't move, and the salmon swims a certain time away from the smelt and then back. So in that one-hour time, the smelt has floated one mile downstream to the bridge. The river, then, is flowing one mile per hour.

Building Your Mental Aerobics Program

Whether you're augmenting your 14-Day Plan or renewing your Memory Prescription, you can be creative in your daily mental aerobic workout. Just as physical activity can keep your body strong, mental activity can keep your mind sharp and agile. You can readily expand your repertoire with puzzles, games, mazes, and brainteasers from other sources, including magazines, books, and Web sites. In addition to these, you can challenge yourself with a new hobby or by learning a foreign language, or maybe just switching your leisure reading around for a change, for instance from romance novels to mysteries or biographies. Try to pace yourself so that you can build your program slowly, and continue to challenge yourself. Know that you are trying to build brain muscle and keep those neurons young and healthy, and have fun while doing it.

Chapter Six:

Advanced Memory Training

I never forget a face, but in your case I'll be glad to make an exception.
—GROUCHO MARX

I recently attended the Memory International meeting held in London, England. I watched as eight-time world memory champion Dominic O'Brien demonstrated his phenomenal memory skills by rattling off the names of all 300 attendees after merely glancing once at the list. Mr. O'Brien, whose brain is insured for one million pounds, later revealed to me how he accomplished this achievement. What I found most astonishing was that he had simply used easy memory techniques, much like the ones I describe later in this chapter.

There is no magic in learning memory techniques—no such thing as a "photographic memory." There are only people who are really, really good, or "naturals" at using memory techniques. The Memory Prescription is like a crash course—a short-cut route designed to reinforce and build upon the memory techniques that many of us may have picked up naturally over our lifetimes out of necessity, and through trial and error.

And maybe now we are ready for a tune-up, ready perhaps to learn some new memory techniques and get those juices flowing through our neurons in novel ways. And who knows, the World Memory Championship is coming up again, and *somebody* has to win . . .

This chapter will elaborate on several of the techniques you learned in the 14-Day Plan, to help you fine-tune your basic memory skills. Readers wishing to go beyond the basics will learn additional techniques for use at work, school, or social occasions, as well as exercises for improving recall of names, numbers, appointments, and faces.

Memory and cognitive training have been scientifically shown to work for people of any age. The *Journal of the American Medical Association* published a report on the nation's largest study of cognitive training showing that five weeks of training improved memory, concentration, and problem solving skills in people age 65 and older. The training not only improved cognitive abilities, but the improvement lasted for two years. That study's program used exercises and strategies similar to the memory training component of the 14-Day Memory Prescription.

Memory: The Long and Short Term of It

Training your memory means working on two basic functions, learning (getting information into your memory stores) and recall (pulling it out when you want it). Certain brain regions are critical to memory. For example, the front part of the brain, or the prefrontal cortex, controls *working memory*, which is essentially short-term memory. Working memory allows us to keep in mind something that just happened. When you dial 411 and a directory assistance operator tells you a phone number, you may keep repeating it until you have punched it into your phone pad. That's working memory in action, but chances are you will not retain that information an hour later.

As a young man, I was adept at multitasking. I could simultaneously watch TV, chat on the phone, and do a crossword puzzle. But as I got older, I became more vulnerable to distractions. Now if I'm reading a newspaper, the radio may sidetrack me, making it more difficult for me to remember what was in the article. This kind of multitasking interferes with working memory, the memory involved in short-term storage.

The hippocampus, a seahorse-shaped structure in the temporal region of the brain (just below the temples), receives and processes information and, if necessary or desired, passes it on to long-term memory for storage through various methods. My wife's cell phone number is definitely in my long-term memory stores, and my frontal lobe allows me to pull that and many other bits of data out of this deep memory storage area at will.

The exercises and techniques in this chapter will help you with these many different forms of memory—short-term, long-term, and working memory—as well as the basic memory tasks that make it all happen—learning and recall.

Give It Meaning to Make It Memorable

The information you want to commit to memory will get there faster and stay there longer if it has personal meaning to you. A list of random numbers is tough to memorize, even if you repeat it many, many times. But make sense of those random numbers and almost instantly you'll find the task is now doable, even easy with practice.

All memory techniques work better when you attribute meaning to the information. We'll review several techniques to make this easy and natural for you. If you watched a pro football game and knew nothing of the rules of play, you'd be hard-pressed to recall the key plays. Ask a fan what happened, and they'll have no trouble recounting every detail of every play, until it exhausts you both.

Studies using functional MRI scans indicate that such meaning may actually be hard-wired in our brains. If I concentrated on a group of words I understood, as opposed to a string of random letters, my brain activity pattern would be focused in specific brain regions, the frontal and temporal lobes. The more activity observed on my scan, the greater the likelihood that I would remember the words later.

LOOK, SNAP, CONNECT:
Your Major Memory Booster

If you read my previous book, *The Memory Bible,* you were introduced to one of my favorite memory strategies, *LOOK, SNAP, CONNECT.* Here is a recap of those three basic memory skills.

1. LOOK—ACTIVELY OBSERVE WHAT
YOU WANT TO LEARN

The single biggest reason people don't remember is that they don't pay attention. Think about the last few people you ran into today. Can you recall the color of your friend's blouse? Was your boss wearing the blue tie or the red one? Which earrings did your wife wear this morning? Did your son part his hair or spike it today to impress his school buddies? Most people don't notice all the detail so they don't have the information to remember it in the first place.

By merely *choosing* to focus your attention, you can begin to actively observe these and other details. Making a conscious attempt to absorb the information gets you on track to mastering this first memory technique, *LOOK*. Sometimes, just looking or listening carefully is enough to fix the information into your memory stores. Think of your brain as a sponge—you want to absorb as much detail as possible to augment your memory skills.

Slowing down, taking your time, and deciding at the outset that you want to remember something will help with the *LOOK* step. Taking interest often translates into getting involved. I like to use the example of street directions to make this point. If you drive yourself to a new destination by following directions, you'll probably remember how to get there on your own days or even weeks later. If you were merely a passenger on your first trip, you are likely to get lost the first time you go solo. The goal in active observation is to mentally stay in the driver's seat.

LOOK is shorthand for using all five of our senses. Many report that our sense of smell can bring back the most vivid memories. Whenever I smell eucalyptus trees, I recall past summers at a camp I attended as a teenager. The memories seem to be hardwired to feelings I can recall from my youth as well. It is interesting that the brain center that modulates our sense of smell is right next door to the amygdala, a major brain center for emotion. *LOOK*, then, is actually shorthand for all five senses: *LOOK*, *LISTEN*, *FEEL*, *TASTE*, and *SMELL*.

Active Observation Exercises

1. Look around the room and notice a piece of furniture, poster, artwork, telephone, or any object. Stare at the object and try to observe as many details as possible. Then close your eyes and think about these details. Now do this exercise for a second item. Afterward, jot down the names of the two objects you studied. Tomorrow, look at your notes and close your eyes and try to recall as many details as possible (don't cheat by glancing at the item if you are in the same room).

2. Take out several frequently used objects (keys, glasses, hairbrush), place them on a table, and stare at them, one at a time. Notice details that you never noticed before. You will find quite a few—you may even decide to get new glasses because of those tiny scratches on your lens that you never noticed before. (My optometrist loves when I recommend this exercise.)

3. Try to notice an unusual detail about the clothing or accessories or general appearance of the next person you see. Is one button out of place? Haircut very modern or old-fashioned? Shoelace unraveled? Designer handbag actually a good yet obvious knock off?

2. SNAP—CREATE MENTAL SNAPSHOTS OF MEMORIES

See if you can remember the detail of clothing you observed in the last observation exercise. As you try to recall the information, you are probably attempting to recreate the image in your mind's eye. You are already developing the second basic skill—*SNAP*—creating a *mental snapshot* of the information you wish to remember. Transforming information into visual images is one of the most effective ways to fix them into our long-term memory storage.

SNAPs can take two forms, *real* or *imagined*. A *real* SNAP involves active observation, concentrating on what you see, and making a conscious effort to fix the observed image into a mental snapshot. *Imagined SNAPs* are those that you create from your own memories and fantasies, but they still become fixed in your memory as a mental snapshot. Imagined SNAPs can be a fantasy distortion of an image you observe.

Bright, colorful, enhanced snapshots stick best in memory, as do those with movement, three dimensions, and detail. The more vivid and detailed the image, the easier it will be to recall later. The very act of focusing on details helps us to pay better attention and learn the information contained in the image.

Distorting or exaggerating one or more aspects of your SNAPs can also give them personal meaning, making them easier to learn and to recall later. The more vibrantly and creatively we visualize new information for ourselves, the more effectively it will stick in our minds. Exaggeration and playfulness enhance our ability to store and recall.

If I park my car on level 3B of a parking structure, I might visualize *three giant bumblebees* hovering over my car. I have a personal aversion to bees, giving me an extra emotional connection to my SNAP: it would be very unpleasant to approach my car with those three giant bees hovering above it. If I take a mental SNAP of that image, the emotional charge of my mental SNAP helps to fix it in my memory.

You can create a literal image—wherein you write out in your mind the word you wish to remember. Once again parking on level 3B, I might create a three-dimensional, shaded or multi-colored visual image or mental SNAP of the block letters **3B**. I have always done this with difficult names—I ask the person to spell their name, and I actually see the letters as a visual SNAP. For most situations, a symbolic image containing personal or emotional meaning works best.

Mental Snapshot Exercises

1. Start with concrete, real images. Pick up a book, stare at the cover, and then close your eyes. Try to see an image of the book cover in your mind's eye. Open your eyes and try the same exercise with one of your shoes. This time really focus on details before you shut your eyes.

2. For each of the following, create a colorful, vivid, and detailed visual image (e.g., rather than a plain bagel, see a toasted, onion bialy):

   - **Briefcase**
   - **Household pet**
   - **Sports car**

3. Visualize each of the following but alter them slightly so they become unusual in some way (e.g., a dancing fork):

   - **Football**
   - **Rock star**
   - **Orange**

---

3. CONNECT—LINK YOUR MENTAL SNAPSHOTS TOGETHER

Developing techniques to connect mental *SNAPs* together is a basic element of nearly all memory techniques. *CONNECT* is the process of associating two mental *SNAPs* so you can remember the connection later. This basic skill will help you to remember birth dates and the names of employees' spouses, and allow you to never again forget the name connected to the face.

Just as there are several methods of learning and recall, there are various methods of connecting SNAPs. Some people lean toward the visual, others auditory, and some people prefer to create a story to connect their images.

To connect two SNAPs visually, simply create a brand new SNAP that contains both mental images. Several visual techniques can make CON-NECT an extremely effective memory tool:

- Place one image on top of the other
- Make one image rotate or dance around the other
- Have one image crash or penetrate the other
- Merge or melt the images together
- Wrap one image around the other

The 14-Day Memory Prescription includes many exercises to help you perfect this skill. In our research with the brain stress test, we ask volunteers to learn and recall related and unrelated word pairs. A related word pair might be "table-chair." By contrast, unrelated word pairs can be particularly useful as CONNECT exercises because they require mental effort and creativity to come up with a relationship between the two words. For example, the word pair "elephant-window" probably has no obvious relationship, unless of course it reminds you of your pet elephant who you see through the window waving good-bye to you with his trunk when you leave home.

People vary in their connecting styles. At public lectures I often give the audience a word list quiz that includes a banker, a teddy bear, and a cigar. They use LOOK, SNAP, CONNECT to remember the list. Half the audience will see the banker smoking the cigar, while the other half sees the teddy bear lighting up. Whether you're a whimsical or logical connector, the visual snapshots will work to keep the information fixed in your memory stores.

More Connecting Exercises

1. For each of the following word pairs, imagine a situation or an activity that involves the two together. Try to create a situation that is reasonable or logical in some way.

   Lion—Tree

   Paddle—Net

   Cart—Horse

   Cruise ship—Swimming pool

2. Now go back to the word pairs above and imagine a bizarre or illogical linkage for each.

CONNECT is the basis of the link method, which orders items by associating the things-to-be-remembered with each other—the ideas or images become part of a chain, starting with the first item, which is associated with the second, the second with the third, and so forth. When initiating the first link in the chain, be sure that item number one helps you recall your goal or reason for remembering this particular list. When creating a chain of groceries you want to remember to get at the market, you might begin with "buy tomatoes," where the "buy" refers to going to the market, and tomatoes is the first link of the chain of groceries to remember once you go to the grocery store.

Linking often helps when we need to remember a list of unrelated things to do, particularly if writing out the list is inconvenient or impossible, like when you're shopping at the mall, driving on the freeway, or soaking in the bathtub.

If we need to remember a long list of items, the link method becomes a more elaborate method of connecting mental snapshots and becomes a story. The story's flow and visual images provide the cues for retrieving the information. A weakness of the link method is that if we forget one link, we can forget all the information that follows. With the story system, the flow of the story will allow most of the remainder of the list to be retrieved even if one link is broken.

The most effective links or associations are ones we create ourselves, particularly those stemming from our first association. Psychoanalysts have used the method of free association to help people uncover emotionally charged experiences. Often our first association to an idea is the most vivid and can have the strongest emotional charge or personal meaning, making it easiest to remember.

Another application of *CONNECT* is the use of acronyms, or the creation of words from the first letters of items to be remembered. To create an acronym, first think of one word to represent each item to be remembered, and then form a word using the first letter of each word to be remembered. As an example, for the shopping list—*Eggs, Syrup, Lettuce, Melon,* and *Ice*—we might use the first letter of each word—E, S, L, M, and I—to form an acronym. The next step is to write down the letters and play with their order to try to come up with one word or several words. If you can't come up with a word, then try substituting one of the words to be remembered. For the list above, see if you can spell two different words. People who like doing word jumble puzzles enjoy using the acronym memory method.

More Connecting Exercises

1. Think up a story that will connect the following items: orangutan, bridge, picture frame, muffin, trapeze, park. After you complete the next four linking exercises, see if you can recall the items from your story without looking back at this list.

2. Create a single visual image to link each of the following groups of words:

> **Shack—Slinky—Flower**
> **Pencil—Battery—Unicycle**
> **Piano—Saddle—Balloon**
> **Cider—Chart—Apricot**

3. Make a list below of five things you need to do tomorrow and use the story system for the same list.

4. Create a one-word acronym by using the first letter from each of the following items and see if you recall the items tomorrow from the acronym:

> **Eagle**
> **Onion**
> **Tonsil**
> **Necklace**

The more you practice *LOOK, SNAP, CONNECT* to help remember tasks, events, and lists of any type, the more familiar and natural it will become. These three fundamental skills are the building blocks for nearly all memory training techniques.

Remembering Names and Faces

The 14-day Memory Prescription has helped many people with the basic skills for remembering names and faces, which tends to be one of the most common and frustrating forms of forgetfulness that we experience as we age. Often we recognize a person's face, but can't recall their name, especially when we encounter them accidentally, outside of the normal context in which we might see that person. Despite the apparent difficulty of this everyday memory task, you can master it using a simple but systematic approach. You can avoid the next embarrassing moment of not knowing a person's name when you bump into them at a restaurant or party, and enjoy their appreciation for your interest in them.

Let's review once more the strategy for remembering names and faces using *LOOK, SNAP, CONNECT*. First, make sure you consciously *listen* and *observe* the name (*LOOK*). Then, use *SNAP* to create a mental snapshot to help you remember the face and a mental snapshot for the name. Finally, create a snapshot that *CONNECTS* the name *SNAP* with the face *SNAP*.

All names can be categorized into two groups: those that have a meaning and evoke a visual image, and those that don't. The first category includes names that spell out the actual image (e.g., Horn, Carpenter, Gold) or sound like something you can readily visualize (e.g., Katz makes me see cats). If an individual's name elicits an association to a famous person or place, I'll go with that, so my name *SNAP* for Mr. Madison might be Madison Avenue or President Madison. Often a colorful person I know well, rather than a celebrity, comes to mind. When I meet Mr. Jagger, I might associate to the image of my Uncle Mortie Jagger, who was always such a comedian at family gatherings. If Uncle Mortie were not so colorful, I might instead think of musician Mick Jagger, also probably a lot of laughs at family dinners. "Pass the gravy, Uncle Mick."

The tougher names to remember don't immediately bring to mind a visual image, nor do they automatically elicit an association to a celebrity or someone you know. For those names or the syllables and sounds within them, we can substitute names or sounds that do have meaning. By linking these substitute words together, we can create a visual image that works.

I was explaining this technique to someone not long ago, and she thought she could stump me with her last name, *Zamichow*. I paused nervously then with some relief said that to remember her name, I simply see her looking through a *zoom* lens for a close-up shot of her fabulous chicken *chow* mein. When meeting Mrs. *Schurnberger*, you might associate to (the TV commercial showing) someone eating a juicy *burger* with ketchup dripping onto the person's shoes, but in this case, the shoes are black *shiny* ones. Here are a few more examples of complex names that can be transformed into visual images for better recall:

- *Weinberger*: a bottle of *wine* falling on a *burger*
- *Bellenkauf*: a *bell* ringing above someone *coughing*
- *Barancik*: a *barn* with a *chicken* in it

Finally, we need to CONNECT the name to the face. The approach here is to look at the person's face and search for a distinguishing feature, whether it is a pug nose, prominent chin, puffy hair, or large ears. Just pick the first outstanding feature you notice and link it to the name. For example, if Mrs. Beatty has full lips, focus on her mouth to create a memorable face SNAP. Her name SNAP is easy—if you are a movie buff, you'll see the actor/director Warren Beatty. Connect the two snaps in your mind's eye with the image of Warren Beatty kissing her lips.

Sometimes the name and face SNAPs come together seamlessly, without an obvious visual connection. If *Beryl* is pleasingly plump, you might see a *barrel*. And, when searching for a SNAP, the first thing that strikes us about a person may not be what we see but another characteristic, such as their voice or personality. *Claudia* has her head in the *clouds*, which makes a perfect name SNAP for her. The process of thinking up the images and making the connections, or links, will fix them into memory every time.

For practice, let's use LOOK, SNAP, CONNECT to remember the names and faces of the four people on the following page:

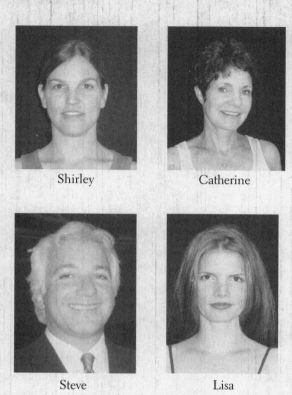

Shirley   Catherine

Steve   Lisa

Here's how I remember them: Shirley has deep set dimples like *Shirley* Temple. For Catherine, notice her Cheshire cat smile, so think of Cheshire *Catherine*. Steve has striking silver hair that reminds me of the actor *Steve* Martin. Remember Lisa by her Mona *Lisa* smile.

Get Organized to Reduce Your Memory Load

Arranging information according to patterns, structures, and groupings can help supercharge your memory power. Many people do this instinctively. If you give them a memory task, they immediately categorize the information or create a structure that gives it meaning and makes it easier to recall. Disorganized people work much harder and usually accomplish much less.

Many accomplished individuals owe a good part of their success to their organizational skills. A CEO of a major corporation most likely needs to understand complex organizational structures and delegate responsibilities. Memory experts use an organization strategy when they *chunk* information by dividing a large group of random items into separate chunks with a common characteristic. I like this approach when I need to run to the market for a few items and I don't have the time to write a list. I'll have more success remembering "two fruits and three vegetables" as opposed to five separate, unrelated groceries.

You can also chunk information into smaller bits that are easier to retain briefly in your working memory, a helpful strategy we all use when the directory assistance operator recites a phone number and we can't write it down. It is easier to remember three chunks of 2 or 3 digit numbers than an entire 7 digit phone number: 815-12-91 instead of 8151291. I might try saying the words *twelve* and *ninety-one* for the last two pairs. Some of us may remember when phone numbers included a word such as "Webster" representing the first three numbers. Those were the days when chunking was built into the system.

Chunking Exercises

1. Group the following 12 items into 3 categories:

Clef	Easel	Clay
Brush	Gift	Note
Bass	Refrain	Elf
Tinsel	Sleigh	Canvas

Without looking at the above list, try to remember the items in each of your categories.

2. Group the following 12 items into 4 categories:

Beanie	Root	Beret
Ground	Barn	Leaf
Tractor	Bark	Cow
Wire	Turban	Outlet

Without referring back to the first list or the list in the exercise above, see if you can remember ALL seven categories.

3. Look up a phone number from your personal phone book and chunk the numbers into groups of 2, 3, and 4.

4. Concentrate while doing this exercise and test yourself an hour later to see how much of the phone number you recall.

Becoming a Memory Pro

The skills we have covered so far should be helpful for typical everyday memory tasks that many of us find more challenging as we age. Some people want to go beyond these basics and learn how to really supercharge their memory ability. As mentioned earlier, individuals with so-called photographic memories, or extraordinary skills for remembering endless amounts of information, get them from exceptional memory techniques. Great memories are made, not born.

One of the most common methods used to really expand memory power is a strategy that is thousands of years old. Ancient Roman orators developed this technique to help them remember long speeches at a time when they did not have the luxury of note cards or teleprompters.

To apply this *Roman Room Method*, first visualize a familiar group of rooms and then, in your mind's eye, take a walk through those rooms. I like to visualize myself taking a walk through my home, starting in the master bedroom, then walking down the hallway, passing the living room, then the dining room, the kitchen, the family room, and so on. I take that mental walk several times so I notice details about each room, which become anchor points for storing information I will choose to remember.

For the items I wish to remember, I place one item in each room in my home. When I want to retrieve the information, I retake my mental walk through the house. When visualizing each item the first time in a particular room, I think of detail and meaning to help anchor it. If I want to remember to bring my tennis racket and buy a birthday gift, I might think of the strings of my old wooden racket that needs restringing, rather than just a generic racket, and place it prominently on my bed. Then I would continue through my rooms and perhaps place my favorite birthday present from last year, in a ribbon and bow, on the living room mantle. This method can be useful for speeches, lectures, or lists.

Now try the Roman Room Method yourself. Pick a familiar group of rooms, probably your home or office, and take the mental walk. Now imagine each of the following objects, one in each of the rooms:

- **Angel holding a spear**
- **Model T Ford**
- **Oysters Rockefeller**
- **Couple waltzing under the moonlight**
- **Burning bush**
- **Mafia don eating grilled quail**
- **Soldier with gory wound**
- **Man wearing a dickey and a gold chain (I loved the sixties)**

These may seem like a random list, but they are substitute images for remembering a bit of trivia that you may or may not wish to know: the U.S. Vice Presidents since 1969 (Spiro Agnew, Gerald Ford, Nelson Rockefeller, Walter Mondale, George Bush, Dan Quayle, Albert Gore, and Richard Cheney).

Memory champs will take this method to its limit when they want to learn and recall much larger amounts of information by familiarizing themselves with 50 to 100 different houses with various rooms in each of them. This method is limited only by your imagination, or the square footage of your castle.

Winning at Card Games and Other Ways to Annoy Your Friends

If you dare to take your memory skills to the next level, then read on. We have reviewed the chunk method to retain a phone number just long enough to punch it into your cell phone. But what if you wish to remember larger numbers for longer time periods? What about applying a method to memorize numbers so you can remember cards when playing hearts, poker, blackjack, or any game of your choice?

The mnemonic method that will allow you to remember numbers and cards is known as the *Peg Method*. Just as a peg is something that pins down or fastens things, this technique helps us to systematically pin down or fasten bits of information. Pegging builds on the linking skills we learned in *LOOK, SNAP, CONNECT* by providing a way to remember items in any order one chooses, as opposed to linking, where we are limited to remembering information in its original sequence.

Although mastering it is a challenge, the Peg Method will forever remove uncertainty about remembering numbers—any sequence of numbers, whether it be phone numbers, combinations, passwords, or social security numbers. You will be able to punch in your credit card number *and* its expiration date without ever removing it from your wallet.

In *The Memory Bible*, I explained the Peg Method for remembering numbers as follows: You need to commit to memory ten specific, simple visual images—one for each of the ten numerical digits. Begin by assigning each of the numbers its own consonant letter of the alphabet that reminds you of that number. For example, I use the letter T to represent the number one (1) because it has *one* down-stroke. I then use this letter to begin a word that invokes a visible image, in this example, a *tie*, and this word "tie" then serves as my *peg* for the number one.

In the following table, I provide a sample peg word for each of the ten digits. If you like, you can learn these words or make up your own peg words based on your first association to the consonant sounds, and write them in your notebook.

NUMBER	WORD	CONSONANT	MEMORY AID
1	Tie	T	Letter with 1 down stroke.
2	Nun	N	Letter with 2 down strokes.
3	Mummy	M	Letter with 3 down strokes.
4	Raisin	R	Last sound of the word "four."
5	Leg	L	Roman numeral for 50 is L.
6	Jet	J	Letter J turned around looks like a 6.
7	Kite	K	K looks like two 7s rotated and glued together.
8	Fork	F	Small case cursive F looks like the number 8.
9	Pot	P	Letter P turned around looks like 9.
0	Zebra	Z	First letter in the word "zero."

In addition to being readily visualized, each of these words leads to distinct images. A raisin is hard to confuse with a mummy, and a pot can be readily distinguished from a fork. Effective peg words also tend to bring to mind many varied details, which lead to more memorable visual images or SNAPs.

For example, if I wish to remember the phone number 555-0217, I would create a story with the following sequence of pegs: leg-leg-leg-zebra-nun-tie-kite. The story might go something like this: My son and I win the three-legged race at the school picnic and get to ride a zebra for the grand prize. We dismount and we see a nun with her hands tied, flying a kite.

That is quite a bizarre sequence of events for one phone number, so you might want to refine your Peg Method a bit. Many memory experts will combine the Peg Method with the Roman Room Method. This will work reasonably well for remembering cards at poker or blackjack, where you'll need to remember at least 52 cards (or more, if several decks are shuffled). For memorizing cards, use visual pegs for the four suits and the 13 separate cards in each suit. In all, you will need to remember a total of 17 pegs (4 suits + 13 cards). For example, the following system creates pegs that sound like the cards or are an image of the card or suit. All you would-be card sharks should now review and memorize the peg word list below.

SAMPLE PEGS	
CARD OR SUIT	PEG
Ace	Ice
Two	Toupee
Three	Thread
Four	Fork
Five	File
Six	Sack

CARD OR SUIT	PEG
Seven	Safe
Eight	Eight ball
Nine	Nail
Ten	Tent
Jack	Car jack
Queen	Queen
King	King
Diamond	Diamond ring
Heart	Valentine
Club	Three-leaf clover
Spade	Spade

To remember the 10 of spades, see a tent in your garden next to the spade you just used to dig up those weeds. The ace of hearts is a valentine with a piece of ice on it. The nine of diamonds is a diamond ring hanging on a nail. The three of clubs is a threaded clover.

Try combining these card pegs with the Roman Room Method by plopping each of these pegs into each room of your house as you walk through when the cards are dealt.

I can see myself now, ready to break out of the pack in a hot game of hearts. My wife plays the two of spades (I see a garden spade wearing a toupee in my dining room). My pal Stuart reluctantly plays the ace of spades (I plop a spade with crushed ice in my hallway). I then smile smugly and dump the queen of spades (a queen sits on my living room couch with a spade on her lap). Stuart may never play hearts with me again.

Advanced Memory Training: A Quick Review

Learn LOOK, SNAP, CONNECT.

LOOK—Actively Observe What You Want to Learn. Slow down, take notice, and focus on what you want to remember. Consciously absorb details and meaning from a new face, event, or conversation.

SNAP—Create Mental Snapshots of Memories. Create a mental snapshot of the visual information you wish to remember. Add details to give the SNAPs personal meaning and make them easier to learn and recall later.

CONNECT—Link Your Mental Snapshots Together. Associate the images-to-be-remembered in a chain, starting with the first image, which is associated with the second, the second with the third, and so forth.

1. *Remember Names and Faces.* Make sure you consciously listen and observe the name (*LOOK*), then *SNAP* a visual image of the name and the face, and finally *CONNECT* the name *SNAP* to the face *SNAP*.

2. *Get Organized.* Look for systematic patterns and groupings to facilitate learning and recall. *Chunk* to reduce memory challenges and make information easier to retain.

3. *Become a Memory Pro.* Pick a familiar group of rooms and, in your mind, place the items to remember at key points or landmarks. Learn a set of visual pegs that help you remember numerical sequences or cards.

Chapter Seven:

Memory Prescription Diet— Eating for Longevity

My doctor told me to stop having intimate dinners for four unless there were three other people present.
— ORSON WELLES

Food—the final frontier. In an adult life stripped of most other vices, discussing, preparing, and eating food has become one of our greatest sources of enjoyment. It can be harder these days to get a seat at a trendy restaurant than a big Broadway show. But meals are more than just the focal point of almost every social gathering; the food we eat can actually protect brain health and boost brainpower. Scientific evidence shows that diet has a profound impact on how our brains age—what's healthy for the heart and body also contributes to brain fitness.

Recent nutritional research has found that those pads of weight many people carry around their abdominal area, affectionately referred to sometimes as love handles, are the most harmful deposits of fat in the body. They secrete hormones that stimulate inflammation that is thought to accelerate brain aging. Studies have also shown that excess pro-inflammatory omega-6 fatty acids from oils such as corn oil, safflower oil, sunflower oil, and soybean oil in processed foods can accelerate brain cell damage with aging.

Dr. Bruce Ames at the University of California provided evidence that ingesting antioxidant-rich foods such as colorful fruits and vegetables, can help prevent the age-associated wear and tear on brain cells known as oxidation. In his laboratory, he showed that preventing such brain damage in experimental animals improves their ability to find their way in a maze, indicating better memory.

The Memory Prescription Diet is based on these and other scientific findings, emphasizing four goals:

1. Moderate our caloric intake.

2. Eat ample portions of omega-3 fatty acids while at the same time reducing our total fats and omega-6 fatty acids.

3. Consume antioxidant-rich foods and provide "insurance" with antioxidant supplements.

4. Eat low glycemic-index carbohydrates.

Our UCLA studies indicate that this diet, combined with the other key elements of the Memory Prescription, makes you feel and look better in just two weeks' time. And the available evidence makes a strong argument that the Memory Prescription Diet, over time, will continue to promote healthy brain and body longevity.

Much like the Mediterranean diet, the Memory Prescription Diet is high in vegetables, legumes, fruits, nuts, and fish, moderate in alcohol consumption, and low in meat and high-fat dairy products. A recent study looking at this kind of diet reported reduced mortality from heart disease and cancer. In this chapter, we'll look at some of the latest scientific evidence, and discuss how to modify the Memory Prescription Diet for specific dietary needs and health conditions.

Bingeing Is Bad for Your Brain

The Memory Prescription Diet includes enough healthy protein and carbohydrates—spaced in small meals throughout the day—to minimize hunger and maximize brain fitness. When we fail to control appetite, especially by indulging in the wrong kinds of foods, we can become overweight. Being overweight or obese increases our risk for high blood pressure or diabetes. These diseases can result in strokes or death of brain tissue, and their end result, memory loss and dementia.

Our eating habits, established during childhood and over decades of social and economic influences, are often tough to change. *Time* magazine (September 15, 2003) reported that in the state of Arkansas, not only are 60 percent of adults overweight or obese, but a quarter of all high school students are overweight or "at risk" as well. That state's health director estimated that type 2 diabetes, formerly known as the adult-onset variety, was up 800 percent in Arkansas children over the past decade.

Nationally, 15 percent of children between the ages of 5 and 19 are overweight—three times as many as twenty years ago—and research suggests that overweight young people have a 70 percent to 80 percent chance of becoming overweight adults. These numbers may have prompted the American Academy of Pediatrics to formally recommend that BMI (body mass index, calculated as weight divided by the square of height) assessments become part of every child's routine annual physical checkup. Physicians compare BMI scores with standardized tables arranged by gender and age, to indicate whether or not an individual might be considered overweight. Most experts agree that in the United States and other Western societies, being overweight or obese is becoming a problem of epidemic proportions.

The Memory Prescription Diet is designed to help people improve their eating habits and make the transition to a healthy brain and body lifestyle as easily as possible. The plan's varied food choices, combinations, and meal plans not only taste good and curb hunger, they satisfy most types of cravings.

Of course, even the biggest "health food nuts" I know go wild sometimes and indulge in some forbidden fruit—filling up on a warm basket of bread and butter before their entree, or going for the crème brûlée when a sorbet would have done just fine. But it's when this overindulging in bad brain foods becomes habitual that we venture into dangerous territory. If you are eating emotionally and finishing whole boxes of cookies or chips when you are nervous and not hungry, you are bingeing. This overload of empty calories can eventually cause oxidative stress to your brain cells, especially when you also are not getting enough fruits and vegetables in your diet. Amazingly, 50 percent of Americans don't eat a piece of fruit all day and 80 percent don't meet the National Cancer Institute guidelines of five to nine servings per day of fruits and vegetables.

The tendency to eat too much of the wrong thing can often be more than just a bad habit, it can be a biological reaction termed "brain bingeing." An area of the brain next door to the hippocampus memory center, the nucleus accumbens, is a mood reward system that is frequently triggered by those very foods we often crave and tend to over-ingest.

Recent studies have explored how taste and craving interact. Study subjects were exposed to the scent of vanilla ice cream and peanut butter separately during a brain scan, and each scent increased activity in a separate brain region. When subjects *ate* vanilla ice cream, the brain activity in the vanilla ice cream area decreased but the activity in the peanut butter area did not. When they *ate* peanut butter, the peanut butter brain region showed decreased activity. These results may help explain why some people tend to eat more than just one dessert if offered a choice, or continue eating past the point of fullness.

This brain region has also been shown to play a key role in modulating drug addiction. Researchers at the University of Wisconsin injected laboratory animals with opiate-like proteins, which stimulate the nucleus accumbens. The animals ended up bingeing on huge amounts of food that they normally decline. Some experts believe this observation may help explain why some of us will binge on fatty and salty foods, even when we're not hungry: the overeating may be a response to a brain neurochemical reaction.

Psychological variables also play a role. We tend to eat salty and savory snacks more frequently in response to stress or anxiety, while sweet creamy foods are preferred for comfort. The emotional triggers to overeating can result in lots of extra calories and weight gain.

Results of recent studies have added Alzheimer's disease to the health risks of carrying extra pounds. Swedish scientists studying the body mass index in adults found that a high BMI is a risk factor for dementia and Alzheimer's disease. In their study, women who developed dementia between ages 79 and 88 were overweight, compared with women who showed normal mental abilities. For every one point increase in BMI at age 70, the risk for Alzheimer's disease increased by 36 percent. The risk was not present for the men in the study.

But hey, fellas, before you go slathering extra cream cheese on that bagel, keep in mind that excess weight might well kill you before you have time to lose your memory abilities. In a 16-year longitudinal study of more than 900,000 Americans, the heaviest people at the onset had death rates from cancer that were 52 percent higher for men and 62 percent higher for women, when compared with men and women with normal body weights for their heights. Two simple lifestyle choices would go a long way to minimize the obesity and overweight epidemic: increased physical activity and a healthy brain diet.

Honey, Does My Brain Look Fat?

The cells of your brain—cells that determine your intelligence, heartbeat, muscular movements, subconscious, and consciousness—are made entirely out of fat. In recent years there has been much focus on the amount of fat we should eat and what form that fat should take. In the 1980s, many people steered their diets toward very low or no-fat foods. However, when you lower a food's fat content, you usually lose taste unless you add sugar. During this era, the food industry came out with thousands of fat-free foods, and in some cases the fat-free foods had *more* calories than the full-fat versions due to added sugar. Studies conducted within that period indicated that the incidence of obesity increased despite the large number of fat-free foods.

Most nutritional authorities are now focusing on the *type* of fats in our food, and emphasizing increased consumption of healthy fats, most of which fall into the category of omega-3 fatty acids. Among the bad fats that we should decrease our intake of are trans-fatty acids, produced during chemical processing. Studies show a link between the amounts of trans-fatty acids ingested and the risk for heart disease. They are also thought to cause inflammation and contribute to brain cell damage as we age.

Other "bad fats" include omega-6 fatty acids, which comprise 60 percent of the total fatty acids in corn oil. Corn oil and other high omega-6 vegetable oils are sprinkled throughout the American food supply in foods such as margarine, mayonnaise, most processed foods, fried foods, and vegetable oils.

Omega-3 fatty acids, or "good fats," are found in plants and fish. They are anti-inflammatory, and thus help protect the heart and the brain.

The Inuit Eskimos of northern Canada and Greenland obtain up to two thirds of daily calories from fat by eating a traditional diet of fish and seal blubber. The high level of omega-3 fats in their fish diet protects them against heart disease. More critical than the exact amount of omega-3 fats in the diet is the need to balance the amount of omega-3 with the amount of omega-6 fats. The traditional Inuit diet contains about 1 portion of omega-3 fat for every 3 portions of omega-6 fat, compared with the typical American diet's one portion of omega-3s for every 20 portions of omega-6s. Traditional healthy diets such as the Mediterranean Diet have a ratio of omega-3 to omega-6 of about 1 to 3. Olive oil has very low levels of omega-6 and is a rich source of monounsaturated fatty acid. While this oil is brain healthy, it still adds calories to the diet, so you have to be careful with how much you add to your foods. Your brain will be happy with olive oil, as it will help keep the ratio of omega-6 to omega-3 fatty acids low, and it is the ratio that is most important in controlling inflammation in the brain.

Several studies have found that people from different parts of the world who eat diets low in animal fat have a lower risk for developing hypertension, high cholesterol, diabetes, and dementia. This is the case for Nigerians who eat diets consisting of yams, palm oil, and a small amount of fish, when compared with African Americans who eat the typical high animal fat American diet.

Some popular high protein/low carbohydrate diets, such as the Atkins Diet, promote a considerable intake of meat and other animal products, which can be very rich in omega-6 fatty acids. The way in which these fats negatively affect brain function is believed to involve a combination of influences on brain circulation, inflammation, and cell development and regeneration.

Dr. Atkins' theory rests on the idea that the body burns carbohydrates before it burns fat, and by limiting carbohydrates, the body is forced into a "ketotic" state, wherein it burns fat for fuel and causes weight loss. Critics point out that by cutting back on whole grains, fruits, and vegetables, the Atkins Diet limits important sources of minerals, vitamins, and fiber, and may negatively affect cholesterol and cardiovascular health.

Diets high in omega-6 fats may contribute to chronic brain inflammation, a possible underlying mechanism in Alzheimer's disease and other neurodegenerative disorders. Omega-6 fatty acids may also impair memory through their effects on the hormone insulin. Laboratory animals that are fed omega-6 fats have greater difficulty learning and getting through mazes. In addition, their brain cells show fewer branches or dendrites.

Eating omega-6 fats also increases risk for insulin resistance—insulin becomes less effective in getting glucose into cells, putting people at greater risk for the memory impairments associated with diabetes. Fortunately, diet-related insulin resistance can be reversed, and controlling diabetes with diet, weight loss, or drugs can improve memory as well as learning ability.

The omega-3 fatty acids reduce the risk for cardiovascular disease and stroke and help to keep brain-cell membranes soft and flexible. Omega-3 fatty acids come from foods such as ocean-caught fish, shrimp, scallops, and lobster. Fruits and vegetables are naturally low in fat, but have a good ratio of omega-6 to omega-3 fatty acids. You can add omega-3 fatty acids by eating foods rich in these fatty acids or you can take fish oil supplement capsules (Chapter 10). The Memory Prescription Diet emphasizes the brain fitness benefits of omega-3 fats. Because we generally get sufficient omega-6 fats in our diet, the challenge is to eat more omega-3s for improved brain and general health.

In general, substituting omega-3 fats for omega-6 fats not only protects the brain, but it can help us to control appetite and lose weight. Doctors Brian Wansink and Lawrence Linder of the University of Illinois performed a study in some very advanced laboratories: two Italian restaurants. Using hidden cameras for several evenings, the scientists observed over 300 diners who were served Italian bread along with either a small dish of olive oil or butter in the same quantity. Diners who were randomly given olive oil for their bread used 26 percent more oil on each piece of bread compared to those who were given block butter, but they ended up eating 23 percent less bread in total. The oil dippers in fact consumed 230 fewer calories on average because they ate less bread. Olive oil tends to be a more satisfying food, thus helping diners to keep their hands away from the bread. In addition to helping curb our appetite, it is much healthier for our brains.

Heavy Metals, Man

Although the high omega-3 content of fish makes it a great brain food, we have to use our heads when it comes to what type and how much of it we can actually eat. There has been much discussion that some types of fish may contain the heavy metal mercury. If one were to over-ingest high mercury-containing fish, the mercury could accumulate in the blood to toxic levels, causing memory impairment, fatigue, hair loss, and other physical symptoms; however, this occurs very rarely.

Mercury is a naturally occurring metal that is also a byproduct of coal-burning power plants, municipal waste-burning facilities, and other industries. When mercury gets into the water supply, it becomes methyl mercury, a form that lingers in fish tissue. Larger fish tend to have high mercury levels from eating the smaller fish, so predators like shark and swordfish have more mercury per ounce than others such as salmon or sole. This doesn't mean you should never eat swordfish again, you just may want to choose other fish more often. Children and pregnant women are the most vulnerable to mercury toxicity, and the U.S. Environmental Protection Agency (EPA) has set guidelines for fish consumption to avoid mercury toxicity.

Salmon, shrimp, clams, oysters, scallops, catfish, flounder, and sole contain lower levels of mercury than other fish (under 0.08 parts per million on average). Swordfish, king mackerel, shark, red snapper, orange roughy, and saltwater or sea bass have much higher levels averaging between 0.48 and 0.97 parts per million.

Tuna is an intermediate heavy metal fish. The average swordfish steak contains six times the amount of mercury as the equivalent portion of tuna. Most people eat tuna from cans, which actually has lower mercury content on average than the fresh or frozen variety. Also, the Food and Drug Administration (FDA) reports that chunk light has less mercury than albacore or white tuna.

In the Memory Prescription Diet, I include enough fish to ensure that you're getting plenty of the brain boosting omega-3 fats, but I also try to limit the amount of fish with high mercury contents. When you renew your prescription beyond the first two weeks, keep in mind the potential for heavy-metal buildup by limiting the types and amounts of high mercury fish in your diet. You can learn more about mercury in fish by checking out the Web sites for the FDA (www.cfsan.fda.gov) or the EPA (www.epa.gov/mercury).

Arresting Free Radicals

Just as an apple turns brown or metal gets rusty from being exposed to air, our bodies are also vulnerable to various atmospheric oxidants, known as *free radicals*. These free radicals are unavoidable because they're everywhere, including our food, water, and air. They also come from within us, as the by-products of our own metabolism. Some experts believe free radicals are the true culprits of aging.

Our body's cells are constantly under attack by these electrically-charged free radicals. These attacks, collectively called *oxidative stress*, can cause cells to lose their structure and function, eventually wearing down their genetic material or DNA. Brain cells, too, can suffer from this oxidative stress. Through the DNA damage, this oxidative stress accelerates brain aging and promotes other age-related diseases like cancer and cataracts.

We can fight this oxidative process by supplementing our diet with *antioxidant* vitamins C and E (Chapter 10). People with low blood levels of these antioxidant vitamins have poorer memory abilities, and studies show that people who take these vitamin supplements have better memory abilities and less cognitive decline. The Memory Prescription Diet includes these daily antioxidant vitamin supplements as insurance, to make doubly sure that our brain cells are protected from free radicals every single day.

Some studies suggest that natural antioxidants in the foods we eat serve a more potent brain protection function. Laboratory animals fed these natural antioxidant foods show better memory ability in finding their way through mazes and other tasks. Other studies have shown that people who get their antioxidants from the food they eat have a lower risk for developing Alzheimer's disease.

The standard measure of a particular food's ability to counteract oxidative stress is known as the "oxygen radical absorbency capacity" or ORAC score. This score can tell us how well a particular food will protect our brain cells from the damage of oxygen radicals or the free radicals. Dr. Jim Joseph and other nutritional experts at the U.S. Department of Agriculture and Tufts University recommend that we each ingest at least 3,500 ORAC units each day, and the Memory Prescription Diet is designed to meet that recommendation. Although we could get that much of an antioxidant boost from just one cup of blueberries, most Americans and Europeans consume only 1,000 ORAC units each day.

To get a better idea of the more potent antioxidant foods, see the table below, adapted from the work of the U.S. Department of Agriculture Research Service in their Food & Nutrition Research Briefs (www.ars.usda.gov/is/np/fnrb/).

THE TOP ANTIOXIDANT FRUITS AND VEGETABLES

FOOD	ANTIOXIDANT POWER
	ORAC Units per 3½ Ounces
Prunes (dried plums)	5,770
Raisins	2,830
Blueberries	2,400
Blackberries	2,040
Cranberries	1,750
Strawberries	1,540
Spinach	1,260
Raspberries	1,230
Brussels sprouts	980
Plums	950
Broccoli florets	890
Beets	840
Avocado	780
Oranges	750
Red grapes	740
Red bell peppers	710
Cherries	670
Kiwi	600
Onions	450
Corn	400
Eggplant	390

People who want to ensure that they get adequate antioxidant foods might keep in mind the following:

- By simply doubling your average fruit and vegetable intake, you can raise your diet's antioxidant power by 25 percent.
- Green tea is an outstanding source of antioxidants that does not have the calories of other high-potency antioxidants like raisins or prunes.
- Tomatoes have high concentrations of a particularly potent antioxidant called lycopene. Eating foods rich in lycopene, such as tomato or V8 juice, can dramatically increase the blood's antioxidant capacity.
- Some studies indicate that frozen strawberries and blueberries have higher antioxidant properties than the fresh versions, so keep these potent antioxidant snacks on ice to boost your brain fitness.

Give Your Brain a Little Sugar

The brain's main energy source is sugar, or glucose, and it gets much of this brain food through the carbohydrates in our diet. Unlike other cells in our bodies, brain cells cannot convert fats or proteins into glucose, so daily dietary sugar is a requirement for optimal functioning. Low blood sugar levels often make a person feel lethargic, irritable, and mentally dull. But give that person a meal, a power bar, or a glass of juice, and watch their mood improve and their concentration abilities return.

Carbohydrates, or starches, are actually simple sugars or long chains of sugar molecules that are linked together, and play a big role in any diet plan. Athletes have been known to "carbo load" when preparing for endurance events such as marathons, and they often drink high-carbohydrate sports drinks during competitive events and intense exercise. Our bodies store carbohydrates as glycogen, and only in very limited amounts. Although glycogen gets used directly by the particular muscle being exercised, once that muscle runs out, it cannot "borrow" from other resting muscles. This glycogen depletion can greatly diminish an athlete's performance.

Many contemporary diets have increased the proportions of carbohydrates. More important than the actual quantity of a carbohydrate is its molecular structure, which determines how rapidly it will be digested and get into the bloodstream.

After eating a meal, our blood sugar level increases, which triggers the pancreas to produce insulin—the hormone that gets glucose into cells where it is needed for energy. Certain carbohydrates cause sharp spikes in blood sugar that overwork the pancreas, which over time can cause the body to become insulin resistant or unable to effectively use insulin. Diabetes, an illness that afflicts 16 million Americans, is essentially insulin resistance. Diabetics develop impaired circulation in the brain, leading to strokes or death of brain tissue and memory loss, and our diet can definitely increase our risk of developing this disease. Studies have shown that eating a healthy diet, losing as few as 10 pounds, and exercising regularly can reduce the risk for developing diabetes by more than 50 percent.

Nutritional scientists have tested different carbohydrates and other foods to determine how rapidly they cause blood sugars to spike. They rate these carbohydrates on a scale known as the *glycemic index*, where 0 is the healthiest brain carbohydrate and 100 the unhealthiest. Eating exclusively carbohydrates with a high glycemic index rating will increase risk for diabetes.

To keep our brains healthy and fit, we need to maintain an even glucose level and avoid blood sugar fluctuations as much as possible. An optimal diet is rich in the carbohydrates that are both slowly absorbed and slowly digested. Starchy foods such as bread, potatoes, and some types of rice are digested and absorbed very quickly. They are considered high glycemic index carbohydrates and can increase hunger and promote overeating and obesity. Surprisingly, foods containing lots of sugar, such as candy and ice cream, do not dramatically increase blood sugar, but instead lead to low or moderate blood sugar responses.

A new study indicates that the link between blood sugar processing problems and memory loss may be more important than previously appreciated. In an article published in the *Proceedings of the National Academy of Sciences*, Dr. Antoinio Convit and colleagues at New York University described how a person's memory abilities can become impaired even before they develop full-blown diabetes. The scientists studied 30 middle-age and older individuals without diabetes and measured how quickly the volunteers metabolized blood sugar after eating a meal.

They found that the slower the volunteers metabolized blood sugar, the worse their memory performance. Brain MRI scans showed that these slow metabolizers also had smaller hippocampal memory centers in their brains. This observation is consistent with the fact that the longer sugar or glucose stays in the bloodstream, the less available it is to fuel the brain's cells. Thus, people who don't process blood sugar in a normal way can develop a prediabetic condition associated with impaired memory and shrinkage of brain memory centers.

Our brains need a steady flow of sugar to keep them optimally fit, and maintaining an even glucose level in the brain and avoiding blood sugar fluctuations should be everyone's goal. We can protect our brains from the onslaught of chronic sugar overload and insulin surges by avoiding high glycemic index foods that cause peaks and valleys in blood sugar levels, and instead eating low glycemic index foods that lead to gradual rises and falls in blood sugar levels.

The Memory Prescription Diet emphasizes these low glycemic index carbs and includes at least five meals daily, making it the kind of diet that maintains steady blood sugar levels in order to lower the risk for developing diabetes. People with diabetes also will find the Prescription diet helpful for keeping their blood sugar in the normal range.

When thinking about our daily diet plans, also keep in mind a few other tips for maintaining blood sugars at a steady level. Fresh fruits and vegetables have low glycemic indexes. Acidic foods like vinegar, lemon juice, and even sourdough breads also tend to slow digestion. Lists like the following can also help us to avoid the high glycemic carbohydrates that unfortunately many of us love and crave. If you need that occasional indulgence of a bad carb fix, be

sure to combine it with a low glycemic index carbohydrate in order to neu-
tralize the blood sugar spike.

HOW MUCH DO SOME COMMON FOODS SPIKE BLOOD SUGAR?

Minimal (Glycemic Index<40)

Apple	Lima beans
Apricots, dried	Nonfat yogurt
Cherries	Peanut M&M's
Fettuccine	Peanuts
Kidney beans	Skim milk
Lentils	Soybeans

Low (Glycemic Index 40–54)

Baked beans	Orange
Bran cereal	Orange juice
Canned chickpeas	Oatmeal
Cooked carrots	Potato chips
Chocolate bar	Spaghetti
Grapes	Unsweetened apple juice

Moderate (Glycemic Index 55–70)

Angel food cake	Natural mueslí cereal
Bananas	Oat bran cereal
Brown rice	Pineapple
Canned corn or beets	Sourdough bread
Croissant	Potatoes

Honey	Whole wheat bread
Ice cream	White bread
High (Glycemic Index 71–84)	
Bagels	Jelly beans
Bran flakes	Pretzels
Cocoa Puffs®	Puffed wheat cereal
Cheerios®	Raisin bran cereal
Corn flakes	Total® cereal
French fries	Vanilla wafers
Maximal (Glycemic Index>85)	
Dried dates	Instant mashed potatoes
French baguettes	Instant rice

Adapted from Brand-Miller et al. *The Glucose Revolution.* Marlow & Co., New York, 1999.

Raising a Glass to Protect the Brain

Most people know about the harmful effects of overdrinking. But a relatively new discovery revealed that there is a mid-range of daily alcohol intake that might protect the brain. A recent investigation confirms earlier reports that up to a few drinks a day may keep the dementia doctor away.

Dr. Kenneth Mukamal and colleagues at the Beth Israel Deaconness Medical Center in Boston reported in the *Journal of the American Medical Association* their study designed to determine the relationship of alcohol consumption and risk of dementia. The scientists followed the study participants for a decade and rated their average weekly alcohol consumption through self-reported intake of beer, wine, and other liquors.

The investigators found a definite relationship between drinking and risk for dementia. Compared with abstinence, a specific range of alcohol consumption was associated with a lower risk for dementia: anywhere from one to six drinks per week. But don't go racing for the bar just yet—for people reporting more than 14 drinks each week, their risk for dementia increased rather than decreased.

Exactly how much and in what manner alcohol diminishes the risk for dementia is not clear-cut. Experts estimate that anywhere from one to two daily drinks will do the trick. The explanation for alcohol's brain protective function may have to do with its effects on strokes, the tissue death resulting from impaired brain circulation that causes memory loss. A recent study found that moderate drinkers who downed one to two glasses of alcohol each day reduced their risk for stroke by 30 percent but more than five drinks per day increased stroke risk by 64 percent when compared with abstention. Fourteen drinks each week may be too much alcohol consumption for some people, so it is important to consult your doctor if you have concerns. Some studies have found that French wine drinkers have a lower risk for dementia, while other research indicates that beer and hard liquor are protective as well. I am not suggesting that you run out and grab a six-pack to protect your brain, but if you already drink alcohol in moderation, the scientific evidence should reassure you that it may help you stay mentally sharp over the years.

Making the Memory Prescription Diet Work for You

Many of us are particular about our food or have special dietary needs. Others may wish to focus their program to address other goals beyond just memory improvement, such as losing weight or keeping blood pressure in a normal range. Here are a few common areas where people might wish to modify their Memory Prescription Diet so it works for them.

LOSING WEIGHT

Nearly two-thirds of U.S. adults are overweight, and many *Memory Prescription* readers may be interested in losing weight. Even without modifying the basic 14-Day Plan, the brain-healthy components of the diet will also help overweight individuals to shed pounds. The ideal body weight tables in Chapter 2 can serve as a general guide to help you decide if losing weight might be good for your brain and body health.

Recent studies have found that five, rather than three, meals each day is associated with a lower risk of obesity, and the Memory Prescription Diet has five daily meals (breakfast, mid-morning snack, lunch, afternoon snack, and dinner) to assist the average dieter. Studies have also found that skipping breakfast is associated with increased risk for obesity, so creating and sticking with the habit of a healthy breakfast is a must for avoiding weight gain. Dining out can make it difficult for some people to stay on their diet, and studies indicate that dining out frequently increases our risk for obesity. Those who cannot resist the inviting breadbaskets and high-calorie desserts might want to minimize their frequency of dining out.

If you think you need to drop a few additional pounds, you may wish to check with your doctor first, especially if you are taking medications or have a chronic medical condition. You might also consider the following strategies:

- **Keep active to burn calories. Try to bump up the physical activity component of your Memory Prescription to a higher level.**
- **Drink plenty of water or seltzer, at least eight glasses a day.**
- **If you get hungry between meals, try more frequent but smaller meals and snacks. Minimizing hunger pangs will help you avoid any junk food binges.**
- **Use spices, herbs, garlic, salsa, and other healthy taste-enhancers to help distract you from the tasty high-calorie treats.**

- Cut down on dining out. When you do eat out, try splitting an entrée with a friend. Don't be modest about special requests (e.g., no cream, butter, etc.).
- When it comes to portions, smaller is better.
- Limit nighttime snacking. Brush your teeth two hours before bedtime as a reminder.
- If you have difficulty kicking the habit of perpetual snacking or grazing, learn to enjoy healthy snacks such as carrots and celery, or try low-cal treats like frozen juice bars.

BUILDING BULK

The portion sizes suggested in the Memory Prescription Diet are intended for the average reader. Although risk of obesity is the concern for many Americans, some people feel they need to add weight. If your body weight falls below the ideal range listed in the tables in Chapter 2, then you may wish to increase the recommended portions in the Prescription Diet. If there has been a sudden change in your body weight or you fall far below the averages, talking with your doctor is an important first step. Low body weight can be a sign of depression, physical illness, or other conditions requiring medical attention. The increased physical fitness activity in the Memory Prescription Plan may help to increase some people's appetites, which in turn may prompt them to increase their meal and snack portion size as needed.

WHAT IF YOU JUST DON'T LIKE FISH?

The Memory Prescription Diet, like many healthy diets, emphasizes fish because of the high amounts of omega-3 fats and low amounts of omega-6 fats. People who don't care for fish can easily modify the diet to include enough protein and omega-3 fatty acids. If you change nothing else about the Memory Prescription Diet other than cutting out the fish and substituting comparable amounts of chicken breast, veal, or other lean meats, you will still get adequate amounts of omega-3 fats through the daily supplements and non-fish sources such as olive oil and nuts. Some people like to sprinkle ground flaxseed on their cereal or yogurt for an extra omega-3 punch. You can also get omega-3 fatty acids from brown rice, Brazil nuts, walnuts, beans, olive oil, tofu, and whole grain breads.

LOWER YOUR BLOOD PRESSURE WHILE YOU EAT

High blood pressure or hypertension is a common condition affecting over half the population by the time they reach age 65. If left unchecked, high blood pressure can lead to strokes that may reduce memory ability. Effective medications are available to treat hypertension but they sometimes have unpleasant side effects. Scientific evidence makes it abundantly clear that merely reducing the amount of salt in our diet can have an important effect on lowering our blood pressure.

A recent large-scale analysis of the available evidence concluded that even a modest reduction in salt intake for just four weeks has a significant effect on blood pressure in people with hypertension or those with normal blood pressure levels. These findings suggest that even healthy people without hypertension will reduce their risk for strokes if they lower their salt intake. Another recent study found that combining a low salt diet with other healthy lifestyle interventions such as physical exercise reduces both blood pressure and risk for future heart disease.

If you have high blood pressure, you can follow the Memory Prescription Diet without any modification, but you need to avoid adding extra salt to your food. Seasoning with lemon juice often helps enhance the flavor of food when salt is used minimally. Even if you don't have hypertension, you might want to consider limiting your use of salt as a preventive measure to avoid future blood pressure issues.

HIGH CHOLESTEROL

High blood cholesterol presents no symptoms, but left untreated for a pro-longed period, high cholesterol can lead to several serious conditions includ-ing atherosclerosis (hardening of the arteries), coronary artery disease, and stroke. Upon diagnosis, unless that person's levels of triglycerides or the harm-ful LDL cholesterol are extremely high, the doctor often recommends begin-ning treatment by diet modification. Cholesterol-rich foods and saturated fats will only increase this harmful LDL cholesterol, while healthier polyunsatu-rated fats, particularly the omega-3 fatty acids, and monounsaturated fats de-crease them. Many individuals will find that their cholesterol levels go down after a few weeks on the Memory Prescription Diet. For all you cholesterol watchers, refer to the following box for a listing of good foods, bad foods, and acceptable foods (in moderation).

Managing Cholesterol:
What Foods to Eat and What to Avoid

Good choices

   Fruits and vegetables (including garlic, ginger)

   Green tea

   Soluble fiber (e.g., oat bran, oatmeal)

   Nuts (e.g., almonds, pecans, walnuts)

   Olive oil

   Fish (e.g., bluefish, herring, salmon, tuna)

OK choices (in moderation)

   Shellfish

   Egg yolks

   Corn oils

Bad choices

Coconut oil

Palm oil

Red meats (e.g., bacon, fatty steaks, hamburger, liver, sausage)

Whole milk

VEGETARIANS

Many people follow a vegetarian diet for health or religious reasons, and it is certainly possible to make substitutions in the Memory Prescription Diet to fit in with a vegetarian's nutritional needs. Some studies suggest that vegetarians have lower rates of heart disease and diabetes, perhaps because of their avoidance of animal fats. But many vegetarians live healthier-than-average lifestyles in general, which could also explain such health benefits.

Vegetarians face the challenge of ingesting enough protein every day. Plant sources of protein, including whole grains, legumes, vegetables, seeds, and nuts, all contain essential and nonessential amino acids and can provide the adequate amounts needed. Soy protein is another popular source. Vegetarians also need to make sure they get sufficient amounts of the basic required nutrients.

A recent Swedish study found that many vegetarians ingest inadequate quantities of riboflavin, vitamin B_{12}, vitamin D, calcium, and selenium. Some of the results showed that intakes of calcium and selenium were too low even with the inclusion of dietary supplements. A particular concern about inadequate intake of vitamin B_{12} is that it can lead to elevated homocysteine levels, which is a known risk factor for brain aging and dementia. The table below indicates several alternative, non-meat sources for some basic required nutrients:

Alternative Sources of Some Basic Nutrients for Vegetarians

Calcium	Kale, green vegetables
Riboflavin, Vitamin B$_3$ complex (niacin)	Cereals, leafy vegetables
Thiamine	Cereals
Iron	Whole grain cereals, nuts, green vegetables (supplements recommended during pregnancy)
Magnesium	Whole grains, green vegetables
Pyridoxin (B$_6$)	Cereals, bananas
Selenium	Whole grains
Vitamins A and K, Folate	Leafy vegetables
Vitamin B$_{12}$	Fortified cereals, soy products
Vitamin D	Sunlight
Zinc	Whole grains, nuts, legumes

More Diet Tips to Keep Your Brain and Body Healthy and Young

SAILING BEYOND WATER

A great way to stay healthy, lose weight, and keep weight off is to make sure you get enough liquids each day. The Memory Prescription Diet certainly pushes water, but some people complain that eight or more glasses of water a day is a bore to pour. Variety seekers will be glad to know that researchers at the University of Nebraska found that other beverages keep us hydrated just as well as water. They put healthy, young, adult volunteers on the same diet, and divided them into groups based on whether they drank water alone or water plus different combinations of beverages, including colas, diet sodas, citrus drinks, and coffee. Slight decreases in body weight were observed in all groups, and the type of beverage made no difference on the amount of body-weight loss or on any of the body hydration measures. These results support the various beverage options suggested in the Memory Prescription Diet.

ALUMINUM ON THE BRAIN

Among the many potential environmental risks for developing Alzheimer's disease is exposure to the nonessential metal aluminum. People are concerned about using aluminum cooking utensils, deodorants, and a variety of aluminum-containing products.

Scientists have studied this possible connection between aluminum exposure and risk for Alzheimer's disease in several ways. In a recently published study that included eight years of follow-up, French scientists found a two-fold increased risk for Alzheimer's disease in geographic areas with higher aluminum concentrations in the drinking water. Other autopsy studies have detected some collections of aluminum in damaged areas of the brains of Alzheimer's patients. The major weakness of these studies is that they do not prove that the aluminum exposure actually causes the brain disease. It is possible that aluminum collects in brain areas after the damage occurs, rather than actually causing the damage.

Although the aluminum/Alzheimer's connection is not certain, many people wish to remain cautious and limit their exposure. Here are some suggestions for those concerned:

- **Drink bottled water made by companies that provide an analysis of the aluminum content. You might also find out from your public water provider the aluminum level**

in the local drinking water. Most commercial water filters do not eliminate aluminum.
- Avoid commercially processed foods that can be
sources of dietary aluminum, such as some cake and
pancake mixes, frozen doughs, and self-rising flour.
Avoid sodium aluminum phosphate, an ingredient in
baking powder.
- Avoid using aluminum utensils in your kitchen.
- Say no to aluminum-containing antacids.
- Take your daily multivitamin. The recommended dietary
allowance of calcium, magnesium, and zinc should help
to protect against aluminum accumulation.

CAFFEINE COUNTING

An estimated 80 percent of the adult population drinks coffee or tea daily,
making caffeine our most commonly used drug. Caffeine also enters our
diet from sources that some people are not aware of, including chocolate
and some sodas. For many people, the challenge is to keep caffeine use at
moderate levels and to avoid fluctuations. In the Memory Prescription
Diet, some caffeine use is an option. For most people, I recommend limiting coffee and other caffeine containing drinks to one or two a day—three
tops.

Caffeine, like so many things in life, isn't all bad. In addition to potentially lowering the risk of some neurodegenerative disorders, caffeine tends
to diminish fatigue, increase alertness and attention, and improve mood. An
occasional study has found that moderate caffeine use may diminish the risk
of dementia or Parkinson's disease; however, the evidence remains inconclusive.

But caffeine also has some risks. It may increase cholesterol levels or risk
of heart attacks, and caffeine use has been associated with urinary bladder
cancer, high blood pressure, and bone thinning from osteoporosis. Acute

caffeine intoxication causes rapid heart rate and can pose health hazards for cardiac patients. Too much caffeine can cause irritability, insomnia, and anxiety.

Because caffeine's effects are short acting, suddenly interrupting the caffeine habit can cause withdrawal symptoms. Headache, fatigue, poor concentration, and depression are common complaints when we (you know who you are) can't get our daily caffeine fix. Caffeine withdrawal usually begins 12 to 24 hours after the last exposure, with symptoms peaking in the first 48 hours but sometimes lasting up to two weeks. If requested, some anesthesiologists will actually add caffeine to a patient's intravenous line during a prolonged surgery, in order to help the patient avoid a caffeine-withdrawal headache and other symptoms during recovery.

Many people are unaware of the actual caffeine content of various foods and drinks. A six-ounce cup of coffee has 100 milligrams of caffeine, whereas a caffeinated soft drink contains 45 milligrams, and some chocolate candy bars have about 20 milligrams. If you are concerned that you are ingesting too much caffeine, here are some suggestions for reducing your daily dose:

- Try a program of gradually diminishing your intake. If you routinely drink four cups of coffee each day, cut back to three and a half cups for several days, then down to three cups for several days, and so forth.
- Start mixing decaf coffee with regular brew.
- Substitute tea for coffee at some meals. A six-ounce cup of tea has 40 milligrams of caffeine compared to the 100 milligrams in a cup of coffee.
- When you have that caffeine urge, drink some water and get active. Take a brisk walk or jog to release the craving anxiety.
- Try not to lower your caffeine dose too quickly. This could result in caffeine withdrawal symptoms (headache,

fatigue, etc.) and make it more difficult to reduce your
daily dose.

CUT OUT THE STRESS EATING

Because of the immediate mental effects of food, particularly some foods like
high glycemic index carbohydrates, many people turn to food to help them
cope with feelings of stress. Although you may be able to drown your troubles
temporarily by burrowing into that bowl of cookies, crackers, or chips, the resulting insulin spikes followed by subsequent blood sugar crashes will leave
you feeling famished and can lead to additional overeating. Controlling anxiety and stress is an important factor of the Memory Prescription, partly because they can have a profound impact on our ability to eat sensibly and
maintain a healthy brain diet.

Although nearly everyone falls into the stress-eating trap at one point or
another, you can follow some practical tips to avoid the habit.

- Eliminate the unhealthy stress trigger-foods from your
  house, car, and office, especially your favorite ones.
- Keep small bags of fresh cut vegetables in convenient
  places where stress eating most often occurs—near the
  kitchen telephone, at the office desk, in the car, etc.
- Avoid processed food snacks. Instead, if you need a
  quick snack, substitute "brain snacks": power bars, sourdough croutons, blueberries, and strawberries.
- Keep bottled water nearby at all times—when stress hits,
  take a swig.
- Set reminders: post a sign in each of your stress eating
  spots (by the kitchen phone, at your desk, maybe as a
  screen-saver) reminding you to "Relax and Eat Healthy."
- When you catch yourself in a stress-eating mode, put
  yourself on pause: take a deep breath, toss out that

cookie or doughnut, take a break from the stressful situation, and try some stretching.

- Develop other skills to reduce stress by reviewing Chapter 8.

WHEN IN DOUBT, GO FOR
THE BRAIN FOOD ALTERNATIVE

Staying on the Memory Prescription Diet can be an additional challenge when we travel, feel overworked, or are unable to micromanage our own cuisines. The following table might be worth keeping handy to remind you of some foods to choose and others to avoid, for maintaining brain fitness.

SOME FOODS THAT HELP OR HINDER BRAIN FITNESS	
Choose these healthy brain foods . . .	*Avoid these brain aging foods . . .*
Almonds	Bagels
Chicken breast	Cake
Fruits (avocados, berries, cherries, citrus, pears, melons, tomatoes)	Candy
	Chinese food
Fish and shellfish	Cookies
Low-fat cottage cheese	Corn
Non-fat milk	Doughnuts
Oatmeal (non-instant)	Fast food
Olive oil (extra virgin)	Ice cream
Turkey	Instant rice
Yogurt	Muffins

Choose these healthy brain foods . . .	Avoid these brain aging foods . . .
Vegetables (asparagus, beans, broccoli, cabbage, cauliflower, eggplant, peppers, squash)	Potato chips
	Potatoes
Walnuts	Pretzels
Water (8–10 glasses daily)	Pizza
	Refined sugar

Chapter Eight:

Focus on Stress Reduction

The time to relax is when you don't have time for it.
— SIDNEY J. HARRIS

These days more and more of us complain about feeling "stressed-out." We worry over jobs, family, finances, friends, and a multitude of other real and imagined challenges and problems in our lives. For some, stress takes on a physical meaning. They speak of shortness of breath, sweaty palms, racing heartbeat, constant edginess, or exhaustion. A chronically stressed person risks developing cardiovascular problems, deficits in their immune system and ability to fight off infections and colds, and numerous other stress-associated illnesses, including diabetes, asthma, ulcers, and chronic fatigue syndrome. Even cancer has been linked to stress.

Some people experience stress as an emotional feeling that can range from worry to panic, and even a sense of dread or desperation. Research shows that stress can impede our memory abilities. Left unchecked, chronic stress can accelerate brain aging. This chapter will help you augment the stress-reduction techniques in your program to maximize your benefits.

Stress Responses Come in All Shapes and Forms

In recent years, stress research specialists have introduced the idea of the *allostatic load*, described as the cumulative wear and tear of life. *Allostasis* is the process our bodies undertake (stress hormone secretion, etc.) to keep things stable in the face of change, allowing us to have enough energy to cope with the challenge at hand. Dr. Bruce McEwen of Rockefeller University notes, for example, that the body's allostasis process results in higher levels of stress hormones in the early mornings when we are forced to face the first major trauma of the day: waking up. (This may not apply to those cheery and perky early risers out there—you know who you are!)

Our bodies respond and adapt to stress automatically, by releasing stress hormones like adrenaline into our bloodstreams to give us an extra rush of strength and energy to either confront an immediate danger or escape from it. These stress hormones cause a temporary quickening of our heart and breathing rates and a rise in our blood pressure. The net result is more blood and oxygen to the heart, muscles, and brain. Muscles throughout the body tense in preparation for action, mental alertness increases, and sensory organs become more sensitive. At the same time, less blood goes to the digestive tract, kidneys, liver, and skin, since those organs will most likely not be called into action during a crisis or battle. The levels of sugar, fat, and cholesterol in the bloodstream increase, allowing for additional energy, and platelets and blood-clotting factors rise to prevent bleeding in case of injury. All these automatic physiological changes are meant to help us adapt to the acute situation our bodies believe to be at hand.

This genetically programmed "fight or flight" response must have helped our caveman ancestors deal with typical stressful situations of their day. However, we are not often attacked by another caveman wishing to steal our food or take over our fancy, remodeled cave. We can't just choose to fight him off or make a run for it, depending on who has the bigger club.

Unlike our prehistoric ancestors, much of the stress we experience today is not in response to real, acute threats, but results from enduring stressful situations that often have no rapid resolutions—an overbearing in-law, a rebellious teenager, a demanding boss, or perhaps a sliding stock market. In the face of constant or repeated mental stressors, the body's allostatic stress response occurs but does not result in us either racing from the situation or attacking it head on.

Chronic mental stress still causes stress hormones to be released, only these hormones may be flowing continually, without enough letup to allow the body to reset and recover to normal. Thus, the physical stress responses—increased blood sugar, fat, and cholesterol levels; tensed muscles; raised blood pressure; decreased circulation to internal organs; etc.—linger on without resolution, until the next surge of stress hormones starts the cycle all over. Over time, this pattern can lead to a chronic stress syndrome that causes wear and tear on our brains and bodies, often leading to illness and memory loss. The system, in a sense, breaks down. This is what McEwen and others describe as the allostatic load, the damage from a malfunctioning stress response.

It's a big year for Beth. Not because she's turning 50 at the end of it—she doesn't believe numbers really mean anything. But her son Mat is about to leave home for college and her daughter Karen's wedding is three weeks away.

Lately, when Beth isn't forcing herself to concentrate on her radio sales job, she's obsessively making lists of things she has to do. Even her lists need lists. How much wine for the rehearsal dinner? How many sheets for Mat's dorm room? Red or white? (The wine, not the sheets.) Seating charts, class schedules, gym socks, flower arrangements, and so on. The details are endless, and she's on the phone every night until 9:00. Her husband, Michael, offers to help, but it's easier just to do it herself. She's barely servicing her clients at work, and now an associate is leaving and Beth volunteers to take on his accounts as well.

Preparing to leave for work early, Beth chugs some medicine to stop a nagging cough she's had for the last month. She puts on mascara while blow-drying her hair and tells Michael to order dinner in again. She's got appointments with clients all day, then she's meeting Karen at the florist at six. He offers to take Karen to the florist so Beth can come home and relax, but Beth just laughs. She doesn't remember the meaning of relax. Michael asks if she's thought about that trip to the Bahamas for her fiftieth. Beth explodes—she's told him a hundred times she doesn't care about her birthday! Fifty is just a number and it doesn't mean she's old! Michael backs off—Okay. He'll just pick up pizza after work and come home a little early.

Beth is already late for her 4:00 meeting with two new clients. Halfway out the office door, the wedding caterer calls and begins to describe the minutiae of macadamia-encrusted sea bass. Finally cutting him off, she jumps in the SUV and races downtown. Realizing she forgot her presentation folder on the bedroom dresser, Beth calls home to see if anyone is there. Michael answers and she's frantic—"Can you find it? Can you bring it?" He doesn't find it, but he thinks he saw her take it to work that morning. She tells him to hold on and she'll call her assistant. She rummages through her purse, finally turning it upside down. "Michael, my phone is gone! I'm losing everything! I'm cracking up!" Michael yells, "Pull over, Beth! You're going to get in an accident." Beth says, "Okay, call me right back and let it ring until I find it." As she pushes END on her *cell phone*, she realizes her blunder . . .

I have seen many busy patients like Beth who worry that their memory is suddenly changing and their lives are falling apart. After discussing their situations, I often find that besides the big events—a daughter's wedding, a son starting college—they are often experiencing additional concealed stressors that they may not be taking into account—turning 50, facing an empty nest, etc. This type of subliminal or "hidden" stress can also manifest itself in chronic physical and/or mental symptoms.

Beth is clearly a multitasker and has not developed a repertoire of stress-reduction techniques. She can generally get by until one or two major life-altering events make her dysfunctional coping skills break down. Her chronic cough may have been a sign of stress-effects on her immune system. Although Beth and Michael later laughed about the "missing phone" event, it highlights how stress can be such a distraction that it can sabotage not just our memory ability, but also our consciousness of the moment.

If Beth were my patient, I would suggest she reduce her habit of multi-tasking by learning to complete one task before beginning a new one. This intervention alone would have a major impact on her memory complaints. She could also begin delegating tasks, errands, and decisions to others whom she trusts. I would propose she develop more realistic expectations of her-self—with all the demands Beth currently has on her time, perhaps another associate could have picked up the extra accounts at the office.

Stress Is Not Healthy for Brains and Other Living Things

Stress and the hormones that go with it interfere with our ability to learn and recall information. Scientists studying eyewitness memory accounts—information recalled during stress-induced adrenaline episodes—found that what people consciously observe can differ dramatically from what has actually occurred. We are frequently distracted by the drama of these situations and may not even see the details in the first place. Eyewitnesses often fill in information gaps later, while truly believing that those details came from their original memories of the events.

Under prolonged periods, stress hormones can do more than just distort our recall; they threaten long-term brain health and memory function, as well as our overall health and longevity. Dr. Robert Sapolsky at Stanford University has reported the remarkable finding that constant stress literally shrinks a key memory center of the brain. His studies have shown that small laboratory animals exposed to chronic stress have fewer brain cells in the hippocampus, a seahorse-shaped structure involved in memory and learning located in the area of the brain beneath the temples. Dr. James McGough of the University of California at Irvine found that corticosterone, a hormone released by severe stress, anxiety, or even a physical blow to the body, blocks the ability of lab animals to retrieve information stored in their long-term memory.

In human studies, Dr. John Newcomer of Washington University School of Medicine in St. Louis found that just a few days of exposure to high levels of the stress hormone cortisol decreases memory performance scores. The high-dose cortisol level was comparable to what a person would experience after a major illness or surgery. The good news is that a week after the experiment, their memory performance returned to normal.

People who have experienced severe and extraordinarily stressful situations for an extended period have shown greater memory difficulties following that stress, even decades later. A recent study of Holocaust survivors with post-traumatic stress disorder found a higher-than-normal level of impaired recall abilities—worsening with the age of the survivor—suggesting that extended acute stress may accelerate age-related memory loss. Many memory researchers are convinced that exposure to even low levels of stress and stress hormones over prolonged periods accelerates brain aging and the age-related memory decline associated with it.

Recent studies show that chronic stress weakens the immune system, putting people at greater risk of disease and premature aging. By looking at older adults who have experienced prolonged stress, researchers at Ohio State University and the University of North Carolina at Chapel Hill identified unusually high levels of a protein in the body called interleukin-6, or IL-6, which normally triggers inflammation to help fight infection. High levels of IL-6 have been associated with cardiovascular disease, arthritis, osteoporosis, depression, type 2 diabetes, and some cancers.

Blowing Off Steam to Protect Your Brain

For many people, stress is an emotional pressure cooker, amplifying feelings we may already be having or might possibly be suppressing. The way we deal with emotions such as sadness, anger, apprehension, etc., can have a major impact on our mental and physical health.

Almost everyone experiences anger from time to time, and it is an appropriate response to some stressful situations. It often helps us resolve conflicts, but anger can lead to high levels of stress hormones, anxiety, depression, and even memory loss. Chronic anger arouses the nervous system and increases heart rate and blood pressure. Expressing every angry feeling or emotion that comes to mind can be socially alienating, and people who tend to get angry quickly with little or no provocation have a greater risk for heart disease than those with calmer temperaments.

Dr. David Shapiro and his associates at the University of California at Los Angeles found a clear relationship between levels of stress-related emotions such as anger, and blood pressure: the stronger the emotion, the higher the blood pressure. And as blood pressure increases, so does the risk for strokes, dementia, and memory loss.

Although studies show that control of angry outbursts might benefit physical and mental health, too much anger suppression may increase blood pressure levels. New research suggests that an intermediate level of anger expression, somewhere between unbridled outbursts and complete containment, may be the healthiest response, allowing a certain amount of stress release without blowing our tops. Anger modulation is the goal—striving for a healthy expression of angry feelings in the right situation.

Dr. Patricia Eng and her coworkers at Harvard Medical School studied over 23,000 men, age 50 to 85 years, using a standard anger expression scale. Their questionnaire covered a variety of ways people express anger, such as the rate the volunteers slammed doors, made sarcastic remarks, or lost their tempers. Men with moderate levels of anger expression had a lower risk of heart attacks compared with those who tended to express fewer angry feelings. A little bit of anger expressed directly rather than indirectly seems to protect the brain as well as the heart. Also, subjects in this study who responded directly by saying, "Yes, I express my anger," rather than hedging with something like "Sometimes I say nasty things" or "I might make some sarcastic remarks" showed a significantly lower risk for developing a stroke, which often causes long-lasting memory impairment.

Anger, stress related or otherwise, is sometimes the flip side of sadness. In fact, some psychoanalysts describe depression and sadness as "anger turned against the self." Many people have found that their anger may be masking underlying feelings of sadness or disappointment, and I've heard it said that it's easier to feel mad than sad. The idea of modulating angry feelings applies to unhappy ones as well, and talking with friends or a professional is a good option to keep in mind.

Don't Stress Out—We Can Fight Back

Dr. James Blumenthal and his group at Duke University studied 94 men with established coronary artery disease to see which would improve their health more: teaching them stress-management strategies, or introducing them to an aerobic exercise program. The study volunteers were broken into three groups who received either a 90-minute weekly stress-management class, a regular aerobic exercise program, or simply the usual medical treatment. After the four-month intervention period, they followed these volunteers annually for five years.

Those who took the stress-management classes acquired specific skills on how to handle their reactions to stressful situations. They learned to better monitor and better interpret any automatic, sometimes irrational thoughts that stem from stress. They also learned to use progressive muscle relaxation techniques and related strategies.

After just those four months of stress-management instruction, these volunteers showed significantly reduced rates of heart attacks and other cardiac events, and the investigators continued to observe this improved health outcome throughout the next five years. Although aerobic exercise has a definite and proven benefit on cardiac health, the group that focused on stress management fared better in controlling the progression of heart disease.

A study that included over 1,700 older volunteers found a clear and significant relationship between the level of leisure activity and risk for Alzheimer's disease. However, measuring leisure activity in general may oversimplify the effect. This study found that the effect of leisure behavior on lowering the risk for dementia was heightened when those leisure activities involved mental effort, including board games, reading, playing a musical instrument, and other forms of mental aerobics. These kinds of activities probably promote brain fitness through two simultaneous mechanisms: stress release and mental stimulation.

Studies on meditation and other relaxation techniques show that real physiological changes can occur. Besides providing psychological benefits such as reducing anger, anxiety, and other symptoms of stress, regular meditation can lower blood pressure, and heart and respiratory rates, as well as boost our immune response. Meditation has also been effectively used for pain relief.

A study using functional MRI scans on highly trained Sikhs while they meditated, showed characteristic shifts in brain blood-flow patterns compared to when the Sikhs simply recited common words to themselves. Dr. Solomon Snyder, of Johns Hopkins Medical School, believes these meditation effects result from an increase in the brain's level of the calming neurotransmitter serotonin.

When we decide, or *choose*, to get relaxed, we can actually make a difference in our brain biology and overall memory fitness.

Stressing Stress Reduction in Your Memory Prescription

Whether you're a busy executive, a multitasking homemaker, a full-time student with a part-time job, an over-achieving retiree, or anyone with a high-stress life style, you may want to modify your memory fitness program to emphasize stress reduction techniques and strategies. You may wish to do this before beginning the 14-Day Memory Prescription, or you can do it anytime you renew your prescription beyond the first two weeks. If you score above 80 on the Stress Level Questionnaire (Chapter 2), then stress reduction should be an important plan modification for you.

To help you decide which stress-reduction technique or combination of techniques to integrate into your program, begin by reviewing the various methods of stress reduction that follow in this chapter. Choose several that you think may appeal to you because not all of them will necessarily work into your schedule. For example, many people may not have the time to get to a Pilates studio two or three times a week, but could easily take a few moments out of their work day to sit quietly and breathe deeply.

To begin, I suggest adding just one stress-reduction exercise each day and then gradually build up a repertoire that suits your personal taste. If your day is already jam-packed, but stress is a strong Big 4 factor for you, reduce the time spent on some of your mental aerobics exercises to allow more time for stress reduction.

Many of the strategies for reducing stress involve some type of physical activity, such as yoga, jogging, Pilates, tai chi, or walking. These kinds of activities take advantage of the synergy between physical stress reduction and conditioning (see Chapter 9). Other techniques aim to induce the relaxation response through meditation, breathing exercises, guided imagery, self-hypnosis, or massage.

Another route to relaxation involves a cognitive approach to reducing stress through anger management, psychotherapy, and other practical strategies such as balancing your work and leisure, and spending time with friends. The suggested stress-reduction methods that follow are meant to augment the basic stress-release exercises in the 14-Day Plan.

A GOOD NIGHT'S SLEEP

Sleep deprivation has long been known to cause stress and memory impairment. If it becomes chronic, it can also lead to illness, injury, and depression.

For many people, today's lifestyles full of burgeoning errands, heavy workloads, and countless responsibilities can become overwhelming, leading to stress and worry. A large proportion of such worriers find their concerns spilling into nighttime, when they may spend hours mulling over details, and become unable to fall asleep. Unresolved problems in people's lives sometimes mushroom into depression, which often causes them to awaken in the middle of the night or extremely early in the morning. Still others have trouble sleeping because of physical illness or medication side effects. Whether caused by anxiety, depression, or a medical condition, chronic insomnia affects an estimated 100 million Americans.

Research shows that the average person needs about seven to eight hours of sleep each night, although our need for sleep does diminish with age. Without adequate sleep, we often lack energy and motivation, and may feel "fuzzy headed" or confused the next day. Sufficient sleep is necessary for normal brain development in babies and children, and in studies of laboratory animals, it enhances the connections between brain cells.

In a recent study, Dr. Hans Van Dongen and colleagues at the University of Pennsylvania and Harvard University assigned young adult volunteers to one of four study groups: those who were allowed to sleep up to eight hours, six hours, or four hours each night for a two-week period, and one more group that was deprived of all sleep for three days in a row. All volunteers were constantly monitored in a sleep lab, where they could watch movies, read, and interact with staff, but could not drink caffeine or alcohol.

The investigators found that subjects who slept four to six hours a night for fourteen consecutive days showed significant deficits in memory performance that equaled the deficits of those going without sleep for three consecutive days. While the volunteers felt only slightly sleepy, they were unaware of the extent of their cognitive impairment resulting from the sleep deprivation. Insomnia and fatigue are major sources of stress that can impair concentration and memory. Thankfully, when sleep patterns improve, so do memory and mood.

To achieve maximum brain fitness, we cannot ignore chronic insomnia and the sleep deprivation that can result. For some people, just getting to bed

30 to 60 minutes earlier is enough to make a meaningful difference in allowing them to catch up on a chronically sleep-deprived state. Daytime naps can help as well, but if you sleep more than 30 minutes, you may feel groggy when you awake. Instead, try a 20-minute "power nap" to rejuvenate your brain and body. If you suffer from chronic insomnia, avoid daytime naps altogether, and try the systematic sleep-inducement program that I introduced in *The Memory Bible* (see box). Chronic insomnia may be a symptom of depression or some other medical condition, so consult your physician if a sleep-inducement program is ineffective.

Beat Insomnia at Its Own Game
A Systematic Approach to Sleep Inducement

1. What to avoid:

   - **Daytime naps**
   - **Evening liquids**
   - **Exercise or excitement an hour before bedtime**

2. Begin your sleep-inducement program on a weekend, preferably a Friday night.

3. Get into bed the same time each evening. Once in bed, do not watch TV or eat or even read a book—just turn out the light, get yourself in a comfortable position, and relax (see relaxation exercises, pages 206–208).

4. If you are not asleep after 20 minutes, get out of bed and do something else—watch TV, listen to music, or read a book.

5. Once you begin feeling tired, go back to steps 3 and 4 above: go to bed, turn out the light, relax. If you're not asleep after 20 minutes, get out of bed and do something else.

> **6.** Do not worry if you spend a good part of the night out of bed. A key step to the program is avoiding naps the next day. If you can manage to stay awake the next day, you will likely conquer your chronic insomnia in just a few days. The next night, your fatigue will kick in at bedtime (make sure it is a consistent time). Go back to steps 3 and 4 and continue to avoid daytime naps.

GETTING PHYSICAL TO RELEASE STRESS

Physical aerobic conditioning not only improves memory function but it can also reduce stress through its release of endorphins, the body's natural antidepressant hormone. Reaching a satisfying aerobic workout—that threshold when you break into a sweat—can help dissipate excess "stress energy." A brisk walk or swim will do much more to reduce your stress levels and keep your brain and body young than the coffee-Danish-cigarette break or a six-pack after work. You may also respect yourself more in the morning. See Chapter 9 for information on aerobic exercises that help reduce stress.

LET'S GET PHYSICAL, AND MENTAL

Several stress-release activities involve both a mental and physical component. Here are a few of the more popular ones that lower stress levels and promote the relaxation response.

Yoga. Approximately 15 million Americans include some form of yoga in their fitness program. Yoga not only offers a way to build strength, balance, and flexibility, but it can also reduce stress and augment mental clarity. Although yoga can be physically demanding, it mandates that the mind remain clear and focused on the task of staying calm and breathing deeply. Dr. Dean Ornish and coworkers found that 80 percent of the cardiac patients in their experimental group doing yoga along with other lifestyle interventions were able to avoid coronary bypass surgery.

Yoga comes in many shapes and sizes. Ashtanga is perhaps the most intense workout and teaches fluid movement through a series of postures synchronized to breathing. Iyengar involves motionless poses that emphasize posture and form. Kripalu has three stages: poses and breathing, emotional states, and postured movements. Sivananda focuses on breathing, relaxation, meditation, and diet.

Tai Chi. Tai chi chuan is a Chinese conditioning exercise known for its slow and graceful movements. Studies of this traditional exercise have found that it can increase muscle strength and balance and prevent falls in older adults. Studies indicate that tai chi can even improve heart and lung function and reduce stress levels. It is sometimes used to promote recovery and rehabilitation for cardiac patients. Dr. Michael Irwin and his colleagues at the UCLA Neuropsychiatric Institute recently reported that 15 weeks of tai chi helped protect a group of older adults against the shingles virus (the same virus that causes chickenpox), suggesting that the practice may boost immune function.

Chi Gong. Chi Gong is the ancient Chinese practice of healing and energy balancing. Chi Gong means literally "energy cultivation" and refers to exercises designed to improve health and increase the sense of harmony within oneself and in the world. Although not as well known as tai chi in the West, many of the exercises are similar to tai chi exercises and involve common principles related to mental activity, movement, and breathing.

JUST SAY NO TO MULTITASKING

I recently walked into the kitchen, opened the refrigerator door, and was suddenly unable to recall why I'd done that. Sure, I was talking on the cell phone, correcting my son's math homework, and listening for the game to come back on in the den. But standing there, staring at the orange juice and the dill pickles, my mind was a blank and I knew I needed to focus—on one thing and one thing only.

Thanks in part to all the technological wonders that are meant to enhance our efficiency—handheld organizers, wireless e-mail, cell phones with cameras, etc.—many of us have developed a habit of multitasking that can be counterproductive. It distracts us from the tasks that are most important, causes stress, and even contributes to long-term memory loss.

Dr. David Meyer at the University of Michigan and his coworkers have described some of the hidden costs of multitasking. Whether you are jumping from your Web browser to your cell phone or chatting to your friend while driving down the street, you are using the front part of your brain, the executive controller for all you do. This is the part of your brain that determines which of the many tasks are priorities and focuses mental effort on them. Meyer's studies have found that people lose time when they need to switch from one task to another, and the amount of time increases with complex and unfamiliar tasks.

In addition to the loss of time and inefficiencies built into multitasking, the multiple distractions make a serious dent on our ability to learn and recall details. The practice also likely puts our bodies and brains into a stress response, cranking out the hormones that can damage the hippocampus memory centers.

The key to ending multitasking is to develop awareness of the habit. When you notice you're doing it, try to eliminate at least one of the tasks. Make a conscious decision to focus on only one thing. Get into the habit of ignoring distractions, putting them on hold, and completing the priority task at hand.

OTHER PATHS TO THE RELAXATION RESPONSE

Just as our bodies evolved and developed an automatic stress response, we can teach ourselves the *relaxation response*—a state of deep mental and physical relaxation brought on through a variety of activities ranging from singing in the shower to making conscious efforts to become and remain relaxed. Dr. Herbert Benson of Harvard University and others have described the process of how we can reduce stress through this mental and physiological state that results in a sense of well-being, slower heart and breathing rates, lower blood pressure, and reduced muscular tension. The relaxation response, in one form or another, has been used to treat conditions ranging from migraine headache to irritable bowel syndrome.

In the 14-Day Memory Prescription, I introduced several exercises designed to bring about the relaxation response, but you may want to expand your relaxation response repertoire to include some or all of the following.

Meditation. This practice of quieting the mind through deep, continued thought has been around for thousands of years. The popularity of various meditative techniques, both in the East and the West, has spurred scientists to study its physical and mental benefits, and the carefully conducted studies are convincing that it can lead to meaningful physiological changes. In its simplest form, meditation allows the mind to become more calm and focused. It is a process of letting go and allowing your body and mind to be still, without worrying about getting results.

There are many methods of meditation, including focusing the mind on an object, such as a candle, a plant, a word, a sound, or your own breath. Focusing your mind on this object is intended to still other thoughts and feelings. By practicing meditation regularly, the number of random thoughts diminishes, and the mental clarity, peace of mind, and stress reduction benefits of meditation increase.

Self-hypnosis. Many people think of hypnosis as an entertaining distraction at a party or the way to bring out multiple personalities in a made-for-TV movie. In reality, self-hypnosis is an effective method to facilitate a state of concentration and focused attention, brought on through deep relaxation. Hypnosis generally combines deep relaxation with visualization and imagery to induce a trance or hypnotic state, another form of the relaxation response. It is similar to meditation, except that in this state, suggestions are often made to oneself or by a facilitator to reduce pain, diminish impulses, lose weight, or attempt to cure almost any human ill. The success rates of posthypnotic suggestions certainly vary depending on who may be trying to sell you their unique hypnotic intervention. Hypnosis can help reduce stress, which in turn can improve concentration and memory ability.

Biofeedback. Biofeedback is a technique that allows people to mechanically monitor their own physiological responses so that they can learn to control them. People can learn to control heart rate, blood pressure, and even emotional responses.

Biofeedback training has been used to treat irregular heart rhythms, high blood pressure, chronic pain, headaches, and a variety of stress-related conditions. The technique gives people continuous information about physiological processes they normally have no awareness of, like blood pressure or heart rate or muscle tension. Special equipment records these processes and relays the information back to the person through a changing tone or meter reading. With practice, people learn strategies that enable them to achieve voluntary control over the processes involved. For example, you might learn to control your heart rate by adjusting your breathing whenever a light flashes to indicate your heart rate is above a certain level. Understanding that we have this much control over our body's internal functions is empowering, and biofeedback has been used successfully for stress reduction.

Relaxation Exercises

Here are three approaches to stress release that use different ways to get you to the same place: a state of restful relaxation.

- **Self-Hypnosis Sampler.** Sit in a comfortable position, take three long deep breaths, and try to relax your muscles. Focus your attention on a spot on the wall or on a piece of furniture; it could be a desk corner or cabinet door. Try to clear your mind of any thoughts or preoccupations. Concentrate on your focus spot and breathe slowly. Repeatedly tell yourself that the longer you pay full attention to the spot, the deeper will be your sense of relaxation and stress release. Take five minutes your first session and gradually build up to ten-minute sessions.

- *Meditation Vacation.* Sit either in a chair or cross-legged on the floor. Try to keep your back straight and your head, neck, and chest in a line. If you sit on a couple of pillows, it will help keep your knees down and roll your hips slightly forward. Rest your hands on your upper thighs, palms up. Close your eyes and focus inwardly on a spot between your eyebrows. Breathe normally, remaining aware of your breath and focused on that spot. The challenge is to ignore the mind wandering—Did I mail that check? I hate my boss. Who's driving carpool? I'm worried about tomorrow's meeting. . . . If you are thinking, you are not meditating. Even thinking about not thinking is a no-no. You can't stop thoughts from entering your mind, but you can let them sail on by. Don't grab them, consider them, or start problem solving. Simply acknowledge these fleeting thoughts on the outskirts of your mind, like traffic noise, remaining focused on your breathing and the spot behind your eyes. Practice this for five minutes, gradually building to ten as it gets easier.

- *Tighten and Release Muscle Unwinder.* Lie down or sit in a comfortable chair. While the rest of your body remains comfortable and relaxed, slowly clench your right fist as tightly as you can. Focus on the tension in your fist, hand, and forearm. After five seconds, relax your hand and let your fingers and wrist go limp. Notice the contrast between the sensations of tension and relaxation in those muscles. Next, bend your right elbow, tense your biceps muscles, and hold that tension for five seconds. Then let your arm straighten and

> drop gently to your side. Feel the sensation of your
> muscles relaxing. Repeat the exercise for your left side.
> Continue this sequence of tensing and releasing dif-
> ferent muscle groups throughout your body, including
> shoulders, abdomen, buttocks, thighs, and legs.

SOME TREATMENTS CAN BE A TREAT

Other strategies for stress reduction involve physical treatments quite often provided by trained professionals. Although these treatments are often used for pain reduction, particularly musculoskeletal pain, many people gain a heightened sense of relaxation during and following the treatments.

Massage. Massage can be any form of physical therapy that uses pressure, friction, and stroking of the muscles and joints of the body. Studies have demonstrated its benefit in chronic-pain relief, which is known to reduce stress. One of the most popular types, Swedish massage, relaxes muscles by applying pressure to them against deeper muscles and bones. Thai massage includes stretches and gentle pressure to increase flexibility and relieve muscle tension. Myotherapy attempts to alleviate muscle spasms and cramping. The therapist locates "trigger points," or tender areas where muscles have been injured or acquired a recurring spasm that worsens painfully when aggravated. The major goal is to reduce the spasm by inducing new blood flow into the affected area. Acupressure focuses on the meridians of acupuncture, but uses fingers instead of pinpricks (great for all you needle-phobes).

Massage therapy's most well known stress-reduction benefit is its relief of chronic back pain. Most people I have spoken to, stressed out or not, enjoy the physical and mental relaxation benefits of massage, and I often add it to my patients' Memory Prescription for additional stress relief.

Acupuncture. Acupuncture is an ancient Chinese therapy often used to relieve pain and treat stress-related health conditions, including fibromyalgia. Studies indicate that the treatment boosts levels of endorphins, the body's own opiates, which would explain its analgesic effects. Other studies indicate that it can elevate levels of the antidepressant brain-chemical serotonin. People who seek acupuncture and other Eastern medical treatments for various conditions from headaches to gastritis to infertility have reported differing levels of success.

According to its theory, energy, known as *chi*, flows through the body along pathways called *meridians*, and any blockage of this energy causes illness. Traditional Chinese medical practitioners believe acupuncture unblocks and balances the flow of chi, to restore health. During acupuncture, very thin needles are inserted into the skin at specific points or meridians on the body. Some forms of acupuncture use heat, pressure, or a mild electrical current to stimulate the energy at these points, instead of needles. Western medicine practitioner Dr. Hélène Langevin, of the University of Vermont, recently reported that acupuncture points correlate with areas of thick connective tissue, which also contain high concentrations of nerve endings. Systematic studies have shown that acupuncture does decrease stress-related muscular pain. Functional MRI studies also have found that acupuncture modulates brain regions regulating pain and emotion.

KICKING BACK AND OTHER WAYS TO UNWIND

The bottom line is to use whatever strategy, or combination of strategies, that works for you. Many of these approaches can be added on to your basic 14-Day Memory Prescription or perhaps substituted for the basic stress-release exercises in Chapter 3. Here are a few more approaches to stress reduction you may wish to consider.

Anger management. This teaches people how to cope more effectively with feelings of anger, stress, and impatience. Studies show that anger management techniques can not only reduce stress levels, but improve cardiovascular health as well. By learning about our irrational automatic responses to volatile situations, we can react in a more controlled manner. Often, progressive muscle relaxation techniques are included in these courses.

Psychotherapy. Psychotherapy can be any intervention designed to improve a person's mental state, and anger management is one form. Stress, anxiety, panic, worry, and depression are just some of the feelings that can motivate people to seek out a therapist to help them understand and cope with their feelings. Systematic studies of psychotherapy have found significant benefits for many forms of depression and anxiety. Antidepressant or antianxiety medications are usually indicated for the treatment of more severe forms of these conditions. With the assistance of a well-trained and experienced psychotherapist, many people will find that they can gain some distance from their daily stress and achieve control and a sense of well-being.

Put Things in Perspective. Or as my wife would lovingly say, "Get a grip." Sometimes we can put stressful situations into perspective without the help of a psychotherapist. Most of us tend to view stress as external in origin — if only the stock market hadn't crashed or my boss hadn't yelled at me, then I wouldn't be under such stress. But the truth is, most stress is internally driven, based on unrealistic expectations that we have placed upon ourselves.

An effective strategy for putting our lives into perspective is to step back and get a little distance on the stressful situation at hand. This may be as simple as taking a deep breath, walking out of the room, relaxing a moment, and then approaching the task, challenge, or relationship crisis with a fresh start or new angle. Other times, we may need to reevaluate the goal we are attempting and ask ourselves if it is too high, difficult, or perhaps completely out of reach. Setting goals such as these are always frustrating and stressful, as they are ultimately unattainable and lead to failure. When expectations become more reasonable, we gain a sense of control in our lives and we are able to plan and prepare ourselves both physically and psychologically for the task at hand.

Give Yourself a Break. I have found that one of the simplest and most effective ways to cut down on stress is to take a break from it. Parents often use a related strategy when they give "time-outs" to their misbehaving kids. The quiet time seems to calm down both the parent and the child and allows them each to gain more emotional control.

Though a certain amount of stress motivates us to work at our optimum level and get the job done, the key is to find a balance. Taking scheduled breaks is a way to periodically slow down the pace of our inner treadmills and keep us performing at our best. Without such pacing, the healthy stress will eventually become excessive stress or *distress*, and can cause fatigue and ultimately exhaustion.

The 14-Day Memory Prescription includes daily morning, afternoon, and evening stress-release breaks. You can modify your program by lengthening the duration of these breaks, introducing additional stress-release techniques of your choosing, or perhaps substituting the suggestions in the basic program with some of those mentioned in this chapter. Feel free to take an unscheduled stress-release break whenever you feel tension coming on or a stressful situation catches you off guard. Whatever form your stress breaks take—meditation, yoga classes, power naps, walks, and other activities that revive you emotionally and physically—as long as it allows you to lower your stress level, you are likely to reap an increase in productivity and emotional well-being.

All Work and No Play Makes Gary a Dull Doctor. In the United States, on average, we work about three hours longer per week than we did 20 years ago. This adds up to an extra month of work each year. As boomer couples pursue two careers, they find it more and more difficult to spend time together at home, or with friends and family. Also, their personal leisure time becomes even scarcer. Not allowing ourselves time to unwind, relax, and play can lead to high levels of stress. A recent study found that volunteers who gave themselves more leisure activity time had a lower risk for Alzheimer's disease.

I often ask my patients to tally up the hours they spend each week in work-related activities and those they spend in leisure activities, not including sleep. Take a paper and pencil and do the same. If you spend over two-thirds of your week at work or doing work-related activities, you may want to consider shifting the balance more toward leisure. Carve out some extra time to read a book, see a friend, ride a bike, take the kids to the beach, listen to music, or just sack out in a hammock.

There are some people who feel increased stress and anxiety from just thinking about taking more "personal time." Perhaps it makes them feel guilty or selfish, or maybe they get bored and restless when they don't have enough to do. Some may feel undue pressure to take up a hobby or sport they have no real interest in. It isn't necessary to enroll in ceramics class or practice Sivananda yoga during leisure time; simply relaxing and having fun can bring about a relaxed, even exhilarated state that may go a long way to keeping our brains young and healthy and making our lives more satisfying.

Just Chill Out. On a recent Saturday, while running my routine of multiple errands, I stopped at the cleaners and then parked outside my tai chi class. Glancing at my watch, I realized I was 20 minutes early. Having not foreseen this downtime, I had neither my laptop computer nor any handy reading material with me. I considered dashing to the car wash across the street—my car definitely could use the cleaning—but I didn't have enough time before the class started. I decided to just sit down on the curb and do nothing.

It was an exhilarating experience, reminding me of when I was a kid and often wasted lots of time doing just about nothing—pitching pennies against the wall, staring at the clouds, or tapping my shoe in a puddle. This now became a rare moment for me, a busy, over-scheduled baby boomer with never a minute to spare. I felt relaxed and refreshed. Ever since then, I make a concerted effort to just kick back and do nothing on a regular basis.

Ways to Further Minimize Stress in Your Memory Prescription

- Make sure you get enough sleep each night. If needed, try a systematic approach to sleep inducement.
- Get physical to release stress through walking, jogging, swimming, racquet sports, or other activities.
- Try yoga, tai chi, or related exercises that release both physical and mental stress.
- Make a pledge not to multitask as much as possible.

- Consider a program of meditation, self-hypnosis, relaxation exercises, biofeedback, or any activity that teaches you the relaxation response.
- Treat yourself to a professional treatment like massage or acupuncture.
- Consider other approaches that may reduce your stress levels, such as anger management, psychotherapy, getting perspective on stressful situations, avoiding too much work, taking regular breaks, or just kicking back.

Chapter Nine:

Physical Fitness Jump-Start

I exercise almost every day. Almost on Monday, almost on Tuesday,
almost on Wednesday, almost on Thursday . . .
—ANONYMOUS

Becoming physically fit provides a multitude of health benefits and is a key component of the Big 4 (Chapter 1). Most of us know that with good physical conditioning, our respiratory and cardiovascular systems perform more efficiently and we gain greater strength and stamina. Aerobic exercise also causes our bodies to pump out endorphin hormones that produce a transient euphoric feeling, often referred to as a "runner's high."

Working out helps us to control our weight and avoid various memory-impairing illnesses linked to excess body weight, such as diabetes and high blood pressure. People who are fit tend to sleep better and have lower levels of anxiety and depression, as well as a greater handle on the stress in their lives. Exercising can even make cholesterol less dangerous. A recent study found that a moderate exercise program alters the function of the proteins that carry cholesterol in the blood, rendering it less harmful to the heart.

Jumping Jacks Make You Better in Bed

Physical aerobic conditioning can actually improve our sex lives. Over a decade ago, a study of more than 500 middle-aged men found that those who exercised regularly reported more frequent and more satisfying sexual encounters compared with their more sedentary counterparts. A recent study found that the level of sexual activity of middle-aged master swimmers was comparable to that of the average adult 20 to 30 years younger. I have not yet been able to become a master swimmer, but my wife doesn't seem to mind when I beef up my workout schedule.

Of course, the benefits of physical conditioning may require some minor inconveniences such as disciplining yourself to exercise on a regular basis, making time to get to a gym, sports court, or other destination, or perhaps buying proper athletic shoes and equipment. However, in almost every case, the rewards outweigh the sacrifices.

What's Good for Your Body Is Good for Your Brain

The connection between physical fitness and brain health has been firmly established. A convincing body of scientific evidence indicates that regular aerobic conditioning not only improves our memory performance in the short run, it may also delay the rate at which our brains age and even lower our risk for developing Alzheimer's disease.

I find that my patients' incentive to begin and stay on a regular physical fitness program is boosted considerably when they learn of the scientific evidence behind this brain/body connection. I will review some of the most recent findings in this chapter. Also, if your results on the Physical Fitness Questionnaire in Chapter 2 suggest a need to augment the physical activity component of your Memory Prescription, this chapter will show you how.

Pumping Up—Getting That Washboard Brain

Physical exercise improves our overall health and memory performance, and it protects the brain's memory centers through several pathways. The aerobic component of any exercise routine gets the heart pumping faster, the lungs breathing deeper, and, if continued on a regular basis, helps reduce the risk for age-related illnesses like heart attacks and strokes.

Until recently, it was commonly believed that new cell growth in adult brains was impossible. Now, new evidence from several sources contradicts that belief. Neuroscientist Fred Gage and his associates at the Salk Institute in La Jolla, California, found that adult mice exercising regularly on a running wheel developed twice as many new brain cells in the hippocampus compared with mice in standard cages. They believe exercise augments the flow of oxygen and nutrients to brain tissues and/or releases unique growth factors that promote nerve-cell growth in the brain.

Human studies support these findings. Dr. Arthur Kramer's group at the University of Illinois examined the way cardiovascular fitness influences how much the average brain naturally shrinks with age. As predicted, study subjects who participated in more physical conditioning had larger brain volumes than their same-age counterparts.

The brain-protective effects of aerobic conditioning have also been shown in large-scale studies. Dr. Robert Friedland and his colleagues at Case Western Reserve University found that people who had been physically active between the ages of 20 and 60 were three times less likely to suffer from Alzheimer's disease later in life. The benefits are not specific to any particular activity: gardening a few times a week can be as effective as racquetball or daily jogging. Most of us can achieve the significant benefits and improved brain health that physical conditioning provides by simply walking just a half-hour, three times a week.

Research shows that tennis players, runners, and other athletes in their sixties and older have faster mental responses and reaction times than those of non-exercisers of the same age. These older athletes also outperform their less-active counterparts on tests of reasoning, memory, attention, and intelligence. Of course, these studies may also reflect other advantages associated with being physically active, such as a healthy diet, good genetic predisposition, or possible use of anti-inflammatory drugs.

Experiments aimed at determining the immediate effects of physical aerobic conditioning on memory and mental performance show that the greatest immediate benefits involve task solving, or so-called executive control: making plans, scheduling and carrying out activities, coordinating events, and controlling emotional outbursts.

The brain's executive control center rests in the frontal region, considered the most highly evolved brain area, and the area that gradually shrinks in size with age. It is precisely this part of the brain that gets the greatest boost from physical exercise.

Over a six-month period, Dr. Kramer's group studied healthy adults between ages 60 and 75. Half of the volunteers served as a control group that did only stretching and toning exercises, while the other half began an aerobic walking program. The walkers showed superior mental abilities in frontal lobe functioning, performing the various tasks necessary for executive control—monitoring, scheduling, planning, inhibition, and memory. Their improvements in mental attention were particularly striking. In fact, the study showed that just 15 to 20 minutes of walking three times a week was enough to provide significant results.

Weight training is another important aspect of exercise that helps keep our brains and bodies young. Doctors who studied weight training in older adults found that after just three months of pumping iron, older men could double the strength of their quads—the front thigh muscles—and triple the strength of their hamstrings—the back thigh muscles. These older adults not only increased their strength, they dramatically improved their balance in just a few months. Weight training also enlarged their muscles. Increased muscle tissue allows the body's metabolism to function at a higher rate throughout the day, which in turn uses up more calories. The resultant weight control can help prevent physical illnesses related to obesity, including hypertension, stroke, and diabetes, all of which are known to accelerate brain aging.

Getting High on Exercise: It's Still Legal

Evidence shows that a better mood can lead to a better memory. People in good spirits are clearheaded, focused, and open to new sensory input as well as storing that input in short- and long-term memory. Evidence also shows that depression and anxiety can often distract people from learning new information and therefore from recalling it later.

Physical conditioning makes us feel good for several reasons. Firstly, the knowledge that we are improving our overall health and protecting our brains makes most people feel happy with themselves, and many get a psychological boost from the sense of accomplishment and control a regular fitness program can bring. Aerobic exercise stimulates production of endorphins, the morphine-like brain chemicals that trigger feelings of euphoria often referred to as "runner's high." Outdoor workouts in fresh air and sunlight often have an antidepressant effect, especially for people prone to seasonal affective disorder. The social aspects of exercise involving partners or groups, such as tennis, golf, health clubs, walking or hiking with friends, etc., can be fun and enriching. The bottom line is that becoming physically fit enhances how we look, feel, and function, and plays an important role in helping us to live better, longer.

Note to Jane Fonda—Chill Out

During the national high-impact exercise craze of the 1980s, fitness gurus across America coined mantras such as, "no pain, no gain" and "feel the burn." Seemingly intelligent people (I did okay on my medical boards!) were cramming into small workout studios for 90-minute sessions of bashing their vertebrae together and ruining their knees until they sweat off small lap pools and raised their heart rates to hummingbird level. Well, that was then. . . . Many of today's exercise specialists recommend we strive to pass the "talk test," meaning that at the peak of exertion, we are able to talk without straining for breath during exercise. Recent scientific evidence points to safety and moderation as the keys to quality longevity, whether it's diet, mental activity, or, especially, physical activity.

The "no pain, no gain" mantra contradicts my general approach to exercise as we age, when we may become more at risk for injuries or illnesses that might restrict us from the physical activities we most enjoy. Athletes report that simple sports injuries require longer recovery periods at age 40 than they did at age 25.

Realistic goals and moderation in all we do will keep us doing it longer and better, with healthier brains and bodies. Of course, all of us may experience occasional soreness after a particularly strenuous workout such as a long hike, or perhaps one of my wife's high-intensity shopping sprints, but generally, exercise should make us feel *better*, as well as protect our brains.

Steve M. saw the green flash barreling at him at 100 mph. Plunging forward at the last millisecond, he smashed it back with the force of three men. It whipped past his partner and bounced sweetly inside the corner line. There was cheering in the stands. The game was his. The set was his. After six years of whacking balls around these courts eight hours every week, Steve had finally won back the championship of the Westerfield Hills Country Club that he lost five years earlier. His defeated opponent, son-in-law Brad, was sweating more than Steve as he came to shake hands, but Steve's wife Janey got there first. "You were great, honey!" She threw her arms around Steve, but he suddenly yelped in pain and stumbled backward. Janey, frightened, asked, "What's wrong? Are you hurt?"

The next morning, Steve couldn't move his right arm without sharp pain shooting from his shoulder to his thumb. His left knee was swollen and tender and his left hamstring was cramping. He'd been sore, even bruised after rough games in the past, but this time was really bad. He tried not to let on to Janey, but she knew it took a monsoon to keep him out of the office on a Monday. Worried, Janey called Dr. C., an orthopedist friend they knew from college, who told them to come right over.

Dr. C. wrapped an elastic bandage around Steve's

shoulder, "You've got bicipital tendonitis, and the best thing for it is rest, ice, and maybe a little ibuprofen for the pain and swelling."

Steve winced. "But I can still play on Saturday, right?" Dr. C. laughed. "Maybe in three or four Saturdays, and only if you take it easy, champ." Steve argued, "I can't just sit around for three or four weeks. I'll go nuts. I have to play tennis. I need it. It's like a drug I'm addicted to or something." Steve was thinking about how great it was going to be walking through the clubhouse with his picture hanging in the Champion Frame all year and everyone lining up to play him.

"Steve," the doctor said seriously, "you start playing too soon and you could wind up with arthritis, bursitis, infection, all kinds of stuff. Besides, you need to let the cartilage around that knee heal or you could be laid up for months. Maybe have to give up tennis altogether."

"Look, Doc," Steve said calmly, "I'm almost 50 years old and I'm the same weight I was in college. I still run a three-minute mile. I trounce guys half my age on the tennis court every other day, so I think I can recover from a sore shoulder and a little sprained knee before the weekend. Besides, if I don't get my exercise, I get stressed out."

Dr. C. considered, then said, "In about seven to ten days, IF there's no more swelling, you can try some cross training." Steve looked confused. Dr. C. continued, "Other forms of exercise that use your muscles in different ways. You do remember how to swim, don't you?" Steve groaned. Dr. C. wrote on a pad. "The physical therapist will give you more suggestions. You may want to consider some stress reduction techniques to help with those tennis cravings."

After six days of rest and ice, Steve was climbing the walls. When Janey picked him up after work, Steve, still wearing his shoulder splint and knee brace, coerced her into dropping him at the club to watch some friends play tennis. He promised her he wouldn't dare touch a racquet. Janey reluctantly dropped him off, saying she'd be back in 90 minutes.

As soon as Steve entered the club, his spirits rose. He was in his element, with his people, others who loved his drug of choice—tennis. The place was bustling and Steve quickly ducked into the locker room. He yanked off the shoulder splint and knee brace, stashing them in a locker. He stretched his shoulder—it felt pretty good— and his knee was definitely better.

Everyone in the clubhouse cheered and toasted Steve's victory as his large photo smiled down from the Champion Frame. As people filtered outside to the courts, Steve anxiously watched the players. Each time someone asked him to hit a few, he had to go through his song and dance about his shoulder and knee not being 100 percent yet. Everybody was sympathetic, wishing him a quick recovery and all, but Steve felt that some of the guys got a little secret joy out of the champ being sidelined. Or maybe they thought he was over the hill. By the time that snotty new associate at his firm came by and said, "Still on the injured list? Recovery must take longer at your age . . ." Steve couldn't take it anymore. He borrowed a racquet and beat the guy into the ground 6—0.

As Steve limped off the court, his shoulder and back in spasm and his knee on fire, he locked eyes with an angry Janey, waiting by the bleachers. This wasn't going to be pretty.

Steve now has chronic arthritis in his shoulder and

neck. He's had two surgeries to repair the torn cartilage around his knee and has a slight but noticeable limp. His tennis days are over and his other exercise options are more limited than they would have been if he'd waited a few more weeks to play. But the worst part for Steve was, the very next year, a large picture of that snotty new associate smiled down from the Westerfield Hills Country Club's Champion Frame.

In a case like Steve's, I would suggest he try and reset his goals to allow himself to be gratified with more realistic achievements. As we go through life, we may not always run as fast, weigh the same, or play tennis as competitively as we did in college, but exercise continues to play an important role throughout our lives. The key to making the Memory Prescription work for you is to find the right balance of physical conditioning, stress reduction, mental activity, and a healthy brain diet that will give you the most gain without the pain.

How Much Time Is Enough Time?

The Surgeon General of the United States as well as Canada's *Physical Activity Guide to Healthy Active Living* recommends at least 30 minutes of physical activity every other day or, better yet, daily. The good news for those of us who have trouble carving even that amount of time out of our busy schedules is these 30 minutes don't need to be contiguous. New research shows that exercise done in short spurts of approximately 10 minutes can have similar benefits to longer stretches of activity. And studies indicate that three 10-minute aerobic sessions interspersed throughout a day have a fitness impact equivalent to or better than a single 30-minute fitness session.

In the 14-Day Memory Prescription, I have inserted three short aerobic workout breaks throughout each day of the two-week plan, which should be fairly easy to complete for most people. Those readers desiring a more rigorous program can extend the length of the basic program's sessions, or add additional ones as described in this chapter.

The stretches and exercises described in this book are designed to help us avoid injuries so we can maintain our aerobic conditioning for better brain health. Even people with injuries, illnesses, or chronic pain still have several sports and activities available to them. Swimming is an excellent substitute for many people during a recovery, as well as a wonderful sport in its own right. It is low impact and very unlikely to cause injury. Physical therapists or other specialists can be helpful in customizing exercise programs to meet people's needs and promote rapid recovery.

The Memory Prescription Physical Fitness Pump-Up

Despite the wide variety of sports and fitness programs available, many baby boomers still manage to avoid them entirely—they are often too busy with work, carpools, simultaneous child and parent care, and more. Although squeezing a physical fitness routine into an already crowded week is challenging, it can be done, and it should be a priority.

The 14-Day Plan's "Fitness on the Run" segments start you out by popping a bit of exercise into your everyday routine: use the stairs instead of the elevator; take a 10 minute brisk walk instead of another coffee break, etc. Try and come up with two or three of your own Fitness on the Run activities. Perhaps involve a mate or friend in an outdoor activity instead of lounging all Sunday watching sports or a *Twilight Zone* marathon—although there actually may be a certain amount of stress-reduction value in those activities . . .

The key is to blend exercise into your lifestyle and make it a part of your daily routine. Even if you can only spare 10 or 15 minutes a day at first, make the best use of that time and try to do it *every* day.

In Chapter 5, I emphasized the idea of cross-training our brains, or varying our mental aerobics exercise programs to make the most of the time we put in. This idea of cross training originated with physical fitness experts who stated that varying our mode of exercise from day to day will not only keep our bodies in their best condition, but also protect them from the discomfort of overuse of certain muscle groups.

A balanced physical fitness program should include a series of stretching and toning, along with an aerobic component. And it is a good idea to allow for adequate warm-up and cool-down periods. Wearing the proper footwear and clothing will help avoid injury and temperature extremes. Another basic principle is to increase your exercise duration and energy expenditure gradually and progressively over time. The 14-Day Memory Prescription does this for you, but if you choose to augment the physical fitness component of your plan with one or more of the exercises or practices suggested in this chapter, always start slowly and build gradually.

Finding the Right Workout for You

Physical fitness conditioning takes many forms and you need to choose the ones that fit your needs and lifestyle. If you have a green thumb and love working in the garden, evidence tells us that seeding, weeding, and raking may be just as potent a brain-protecting endeavor as walking a mile a day. I encourage people to try several types of exercise and then choose and stick with the most personally satisfying ones. The following are a few examples.

WALKING

Many experts consider brisk walking to be the ideal aerobic activity for people at any age. Walking requires no training or special equipment, and carries very little risk of injury. It is also one of the easiest exercise routines to add to most people's daily schedules, which is why I included it in the 14-Day Plan. You can increase the aerobic challenge of your walks by lengthening the duration or distance covered; or you may want to challenge yourself by walking up and down hills.

JOGGING

This alternative to walking provides a greater aerobic challenge. It can be done almost anywhere and in *almost* any climate, and requires very little special gear other than proper running shoes. People with knee, ankle, or back injuries may want to check with their doctor before beginning a jogging routine as they might have difficulty with this higher-impact exercise.

SWIMMING

Water-fitness buffs swear by this excellent low-impact aerobic conditioning sport. Swimming has long been a favorite alternative to other sports for people who have suffered back, ankle, or knee injuries. Some people claim to dislike the "inconvenience" of getting wet, but most find it a refreshing and exhilarating experience.

RACQUET SPORTS

Tennis and racquetball are popular sports that offer the thrill and satisfaction of a contest, as well as the challenge of improving your skills with practice. For younger adults, injuries are relatively rare, but after years of wear and tear on their joints, some older adults may choose to segue to lower-impact alternatives.

DANCING

Whether it's ballroom, swing, disco, or jitterbug, dancing offers an excellent aerobic workout. The challenge of learning and following new steps also provides additional mental fitness benefits. A recent scientific study found that leisure activities involving mental effort—including several types of dancing—reduced the risk of dementia. When performed regularly and several times each week, dancing was among the leisure activities that showed an advantage for better memory function over time.

PILATES

Pilates is a method of physical movement and exercise designed to stretch, strengthen, and balance the body. Originally developed by Joseph Pilates to rehabilitate injured dancers, the exercise program has taken off in many parts of the world, and with all age groups. Many older adults have embraced a Pilates program to improve their balance and coordination, and to help them avoid falls and injury. Pilates work focuses on strengthening the "powerhouse," or the musculature that connects the abdomen with the lower back and the buttocks. Advocates note improved posture and relief of back and other pain after only weeks of practice. It's best to get started with an instructor at a Pilates studio that has the special equipment needed for the program's unique stretching and toning exercises. Also, many gyms and health clubs now offer Pilates mat-based classes.

OTHER ACTIVITIES

Any form of regular physical activity can help increase brain circulation, reduce stress, and contribute to our overall brain fitness. People who find routine exercises like walking or jogging too boring may prefer activities that engage them mentally, such as gardening or shuffleboard. Still others prefer more competitive or physically challenging sports such as volleyball, power yoga, golf (no cart!), bike riding, cross-country skiing, hiking, martial arts, and so on. Activities that we do with others—tennis, tandem bicycling, or doubles rowing—often increase our enjoyment and keep us interested longer. Chores or physical tasks like vacuuming or shopping have built-in exercise value. (My wife *lives* to vacuum.) Whatever activity or sport you choose, if you enjoy it, you are more likely to go back for more.

Pumping Iron for Brain Health

There's good news and bad news. The bad news: as we age, we tend to lose muscle tissue. By age 70, most of us lose 20 percent of the muscle mass we enjoyed at age 30. For postmenopausal women, it can be even worse. And with less strength and muscle, we tend toward inactivity and increased body fat.

The good news: weight training can counteract this effect. Exercising with free weights or weight machines on a regular basis can slow down, even reverse, the muscle and strength loss associated with aging. Plus you don't have to bench press 300 pounds at Muscle Beach to gain the benefits. In studies, older men using only one- or two-pound dumbbells for regular strength training were able to increase their muscle size and strength by up to 50 percent more than the group that used no weights at all. The weight lifters also suffered fewer falls and injuries during other recreational activities.

Many fitness experts recommend working out with weights at least two to three times a week, with rest days between workout days and alternating muscle groups each day—upper body one day, lower body the next. A typical routine might include a combination of a half-dozen or more exercises for major muscle groups (legs, arms, shoulders, abdomen, etc.). One usually lifts weight in "sets," which may include from 10 to 20 repetitions, and two or three sets are commonly performed each session. It is advisable to always begin with lighter weights and build up slowly to increase strength and avoid injury. Because form and technique are critically important to maximize benefits and avoid injuries, I recommend beginning with an experienced trainer.

Treadmills, Weight Machines, and Other Fitness Gadgets

Some people can afford the time and expense of joining a health club or other fitness center; others prefer working out in their homes, possibly with a home treadmill, stationary bicycle, stair-stepper, or elliptical machine. Still, many others get their workouts outdoors by walking, running, gardening, etc. Whatever keeps you interested and coming back is the right choice for you.

To improve muscle tone and help control body mass and weight, free weights do basically the same job as weight machines. Easier to use at home, free weights can offer additional improvement in coordination and balance, as well as more options for a varied workout. By contrast, weight machines can allow greater control over specific muscle groups. They may also be safer since the range of motion they provide is more controlled.

Watching Your Back

An estimated 80 percent of Americans suffer from intermittent or chronic back pain. As with any chronic pain, the distraction it causes may worsen memory function for the average individual.

For most back sufferers, two major factors contribute: weak abdominal muscles and limited flexibility. Toning and strengthening your abs with sit-ups or other abdominal exercises will certainly help to protect and strengthen your back and surrounding muscles. By adding stretching exercises, your back muscles and the others surrounding it will become more flexible and elongated, protecting you from future injury and pain. Perhaps one reason for the growing popularity of Pilates is its focus on strengthening the "core" muscles, or "powerhouse"—the musculature located deep within the abdominal area, which acts to support the spine and align the body correctly.

Along with an effective strengthening, stretching, and toning routine (see Stretching and Toning discussion below), several other simple interventions can bring great relief to back pain. These include wearing low-heeled shoes, trying to avoid long periods of sitting by walking and stretching at regular intervals, using your knees when lifting heavy objects, and sleeping on your side with a pillow between your knees. Overweight back sufferers may find that shedding a few extra pounds can relieve some of the discomfort.

Knee Keeper

Running and competitive sports can be tough on our knees, which are actually one of the weaker joints in our bodies. The numerous muscles and ligaments surrounding our knees are what really hold them in place and keep them operating correctly. Strengthening the quadriceps muscle and the inner and outer thigh, as well as the smaller muscles and ligaments surrounding the kneecap, protects the area from injury and helps keep the kneecap from sliding out of place. Many other common exercise-related knee problems can be easily corrected by wearing the proper footwear or perhaps shoe inserts. Running or power-walking on hard surfaces such as concrete may contribute to knee problems—dirt and gravel are much softer and preferred by many joggers. If you should experience knee pain while exercising, stop and apply ice as soon as possible. If the discomfort does not improve, consult your doctor.

Brain Safety

Research has shown that when someone experiences a head injury leading to an hour or more of unconsciousness, it increases their risk for developing Alzheimer's disease later in life. For people with the APOE-4 genetic risk for Alzheimer's disease, a severe blow to the head might increase that risk tenfold. Scientists have found that the brains of head-injured patients with the risk gene have greater amounts of amyloid plaque deposition, the insoluble protein that may cause Alzheimer's disease.

We are also now realizing that even much milder bumps to the head can impair memory and accelerate brain aging. People carrying the APOE-4 gene have good reason to avoid sports and occupations that involve a high risk for head injury, such as boxing, football, soccer, racecar driving, movie stunt work, and crash helmet testing.

Head safety should be a consideration in school athletics as well. A recent University of Pittsburgh study found that even a light concussion can cause more serious damage than previously recognized, and any blow to the head that rocks the brain back and forth inside the skull can cause a concussion.

Dr. Erik Matser and his team at St. Anna Hospital in the Netherlands have compared amateur soccer players in their mid-twenties to same-aged swimmers and runners who were less likely to suffer head injuries. Over 30 percent of the soccer players suffered from memory impairments, while less than 10 percent of the swimmers and runners had similar impairments. Although the memory impairments in these athletes were mild, it does raise concern over possible risk for future progressive decline.

When augmenting the physical fitness component of your Memory Prescription, I urge you to consider fitness activities that minimize the risk for head injury. Adopting brain-safe habits such as wearing seat belts and helmets, and selecting a designated driver who is not drinking, will help avoid head trauma and protect your brain from future cognitive decline.

Stretching and Toning for Better Health and Memory

Most people report improved memory and mental focus when they are no longer distracted by chronic pain and stiffness. A regular routine to stretch and tone the body can help people reach that goal. The following are some simple stretching and toning exercises you can use to augment the physical fitness component of your Memory Prescription. Even if you practice only a few of these exercises regularly, you will notice better flexibility and mobility, as they promote your heart and brain circulation and lower your risk for injuries during exercise, and you will probably feel less tense overall. Stretching is a good warm-up and cool-down routine for any sport, aerobic workout, or strength conditioning.

Practice these exercises in a slow and relaxed manner. Repeat the movements only a few times at first, then add more repetitions as your endurance builds over time. If the initial suggested "hold" time for any exercise feels like too much or too little, adjust to suit your own fitness level.

Stretch muscles without bouncing, and never to the point of pain. Some of the following movements require the use of an elastic exercise band of approximately four feet in length, which you can purchase for a few dollars at a local fitness store or pharmacy.

STRETCHING EXERCISES

Back Leg Stretch. Stand about 18 inches away from a wall or closed door and place your hands flat against the wall in front of your shoulders. Lean forward, step your right leg back, and bend your left knee. Keeping that right leg straight, drop the heel toward the ground. Push your chest forward to stretch your right calf and hamstring muscles. (Also notice a nice stretch in the chest.) Hold for a count of 10, keeping both feet pointed forward. Switch leg positions to stretch the left calf and hamstring.

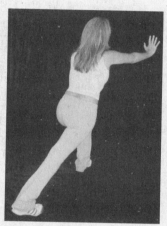

Back Leg Stretch

Quadriceps Stretch. Stand facing a wall or doorway and support yourself with your right hand. Bend your left foot back and hold your ankle with your left hand. Pull that left foot toward your bottom, bringing your knees together. Feel the stretch through the front of your left leg as you keep pulling that foot closer to your bottom and hold for a count of 10. Repeat on the other side.

Hamstring Stretch. Stand a few feet away from a stool or bench. Lift your right knee and place the heel of that foot on the bench. Slowly straighten the right leg, keeping the standing leg straight as well. Leaning forward, take hold of your ankle, gently pulling your torso toward the stretching leg. Hold for a count of 10, and then repeat on other side.

Shoulder Stretch. Reach one straight arm across your chest toward the other shoulder. With the opposite hand, grasp your elbow and pull your arm in as close to your body as possible. Hold for a count of 10, and then stretch the other side.

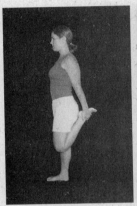 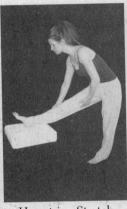 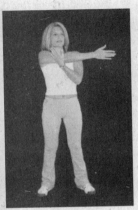

Quadriceps Stretch   Hamstring Stretch   Shoulder Stretch

Triceps Stretch. Raise both arms overhead. Bend the right elbow, dropping the right hand behind your head. Hold the bent right elbow with your left hand and pull it down and back behind your head. Feel the stretch in your right triceps muscle and shoulder. Hold for a count of 10, and then repeat on other side.

Biceps/Chest Stretch. Clasp your hands behind your back. While keeping your chest high, lift your straight arms up behind you. Hold the stretch for 15 sec-

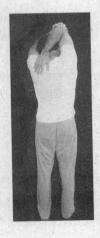

Triceps Stretch

onds, and then repeat. For a greater challenge, bend forward and raise your arms up higher.

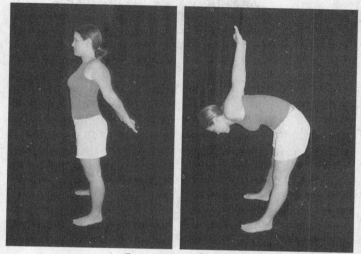

Biceps/Chest Stretch

Elbow/Wrist Stretch. In this age of computers, people seem to be developing more carpal tunnel syndrome and other wrist/hand/elbow maladies. This stretch can help. Hold your right arm straight out in front of you, shoulder height and palm up. With your left hand, grasp your right fingers and pull them back and down. Keep your right elbow straight, and feel the stretch from your wrist to the top of your arm. Hold for a count of 5, and then repeat on opposite side.

Shoulder Roll. Slowly roll your shoulders back in complete circles for five rotations. Now roll them forward for five rotations. Next, turn your chin slowly toward your left shoulder as far as possible and hold it for a count of 5. Slowly change directions, chin to right shoulder, and hold for 5. Finish by repeating shoulder rolls.

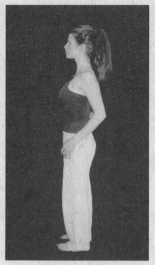

Shoulder Roll

Neck and Shoulder Stretch. Stand tall with arms straight down at your sides. With your left hand, reach behind you and grab your right wrist. Pull your right arm down and across your back, while you drop your right shoulder and tilt your head to the left. Feel the stretch down the right side of your neck, through that shoulder, and down the right arm. Hold for a count of 8 and repeat on the other side.

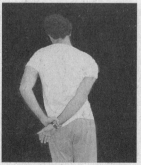

Neck and Shoulder Stretch

Chest Stretch. Stand with your forearms against the wall in a door-jamb or room corner. Lean gently forward until you feel a stretch in the front of your shoulders and chest wall. Hold for a count of 10, then repeat two more times.

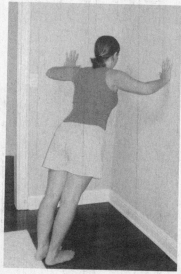

Chest Stretch

Spine Twist. Sit on the floor with legs stretched out in front of you. Lift your left foot and place it outside your right knee. Anchor your right elbow on the outside of your left knee, and twist to look back over your left shoulder, placing your left hand on the floor behind you for balance. Hold and breathe for a count of 8 and feel the stretch in your spine. Come back to neutral position and then repeat on other side.

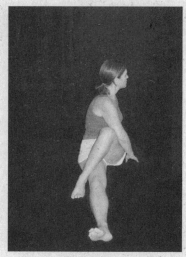

Spine Twist

Upper-Body Floor Stretch. Lie on your stomach with your palms on the floor, under your shoulders. Keeping your pelvis and thighs on the floor, slowly push your shoulders up until your arms are straight. Feel the stretch through your chest, shoulders, and back. Hold for a count of 5, then lower to floor. Repeat two or three times.

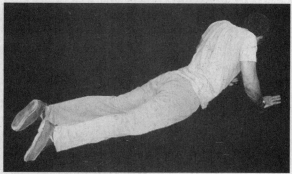

Upper-Body Floor Stretch

Hip and Inner Thigh Stretch. Lie on your back with your legs bent, feet on the floor. Place your left ankle on your right knee. Clasp the back of your right thigh with both hands and gently pull it toward your chest. Press your open left knee down and away with your left elbow. Hold for a count of 10 and repeat on the opposite side. This exercise can be exported from home to office since it can be performed both on the floor as well as in a chair. Sitting straight, place your left ankle on your right knee. With your left hand, gently push down on your left knee and open your pelvis. Hold the stretch for a count of 10 and then repeat on the opposite side.

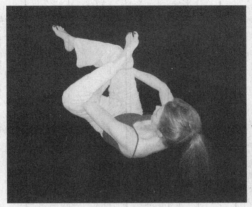

Hip and Inner Thigh Stretch

Lower Back Stretch. Lie on your back with your feet on the floor and knees bent. Lift your right leg and clasp it with both hands. As you pull it to your chest, extend your left leg straight out on the floor. Hold the position for a count of 5. Switch to the other leg, then repeat four times with each leg. Complete the movement by pulling both legs toward your chest simultaneously and hold for a count of 5.

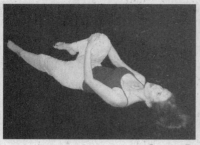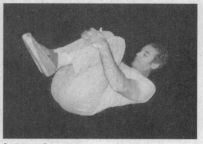

Lower Back Stretch

Cat Stretch. Position yourself on hands and knees on the floor. Keep your belly in as you arch your back up toward the ceiling as high as possible—like a cat stretching—and drop your head. Hold for 2 counts, then slowly raise your head, look upward, and lower your back into a scooped or bowl position for the opposite stretch. Repeat five times, keeping the motions fluid.

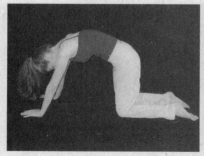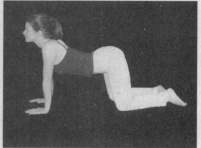

Cat Stretch

Prayer Stretch. With legs bent under you on the floor, reach your arms forward and let your chest touch the floor. Pull back with straight arms while pressing down slightly with your palms. Move your arms to the right so you can lean your torso in the opposite direction to stretch out your left side. Do the same for your right side. Hold each stretch for a count of 10.

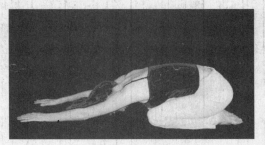

Prayer Stretch

STRENGTHENING EXERCISES

Abdominal Crunch. Lie on your back with your knees bent and feet on the floor. Lace your fingers behind your head, keeping your elbows pointed out. Take a deep breath. As you exhale, raise your upper torso off the floor and pull your navel down toward your spine. Focus on using your lower abdominal muscles without straining your neck. Hold for a count of 2 and then complete a set of 10. Build up to five sets.

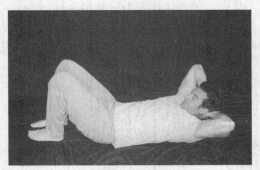

Abdominal Crunch

Abdominal Side Toning. This exercise for toning the lateral abdominal muscles is a modern take on the old-fashioned "bicycle." Lie on your back with hands clasped behind your head. Raise your knees directly above your hips with calves parallel to the ground. Take a deep breath. As you exhale, lift your head, torso, and right elbow toward your left knee, while pushing your right leg out straight. Hold for one count then switch to the other side. Be sure to pull your navel in toward your spine with each exhale and contraction. Do a set of 10 repetitions on each side, increasing the number of sets over time.

Extremity and Torso Strengthener. This exercise strengthens the torso and extremities, and also improves posture and balance. Get on the floor and balance on your hands and the balls of your feet. Keep your arms and legs straight and your body in a straight line (push-up position). Focus on pulling your abdominal muscles in toward your spine. Pushing with your toes, gently rock your body forward and backward. As you gain experience and strength with this exercise, try shifting your weight onto one leg, lifting the opposite leg off the floor and straight up behind you. Hold for a count of 5 and then switch leg positions.

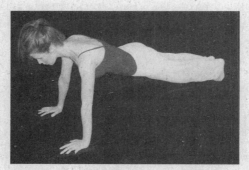

Extremity and Torso Strengthener

Biceps Toning. While standing, take one end of your elastic band in your left hand and step on the other end with your left foot. Brace your left elbow against your side and slowly pull your left forearm toward your shoulder. Move slowly, working against the tension of the band, and do not bend your wrist. Repeat five times, and then switch sides. Build to 12 repetitions per set.

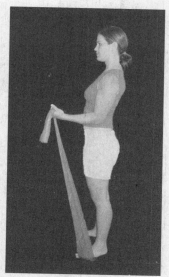

Biceps Toning

Triceps Toning. While holding one end of your strap in your right hand, place that hand behind your head and let the strap hang down behind your back. Take your left hand behind the base of your back and grasp the other end of the strap (Figure 1). Keeping your right elbow near your head, slowly straighten that right arm, pulling against the tension of the strap as your left hand pulls downward on it (Figure 2). Feel the work in your triceps muscles. Repeat five times, and then switch sides. Build to 12 repetitions per set.

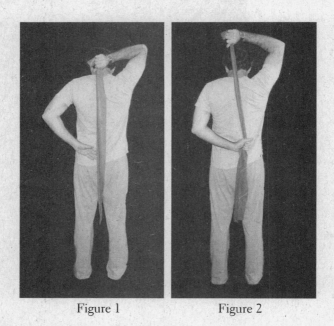

Figure 1   Figure 2

Triceps Toning

Shoulder and Upper Back Toning. While standing, take one end of your elastic band in your left hand and step on the other end with your left foot. Keeping your left arm straight, pull up on the band until your arm reaches a 90-degree angle. Repeat five times, then switch to your right side.

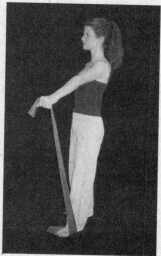

Shoulder and Upper Back Toning

Inner Thigh Toner. Take your elastic band and tie the ends together in a loose knot for wedging between the closed door and frame (Figure 1). Stand up straight and place your right ankle in the band loop. Steady yourself by placing your right hand against the door jamb, and then pull your straight right leg against the tension of the band, slowly crossing it over in front of your left leg (Figure 2). Repeat 10 times and switch legs.

Outer Thigh Toner. Place both feet within the elastic band wedged in the door. Stand with your right side toward the door and steady yourself with your right hand. Slowly push your straightened left leg outward against the tension of the band (Figure 3). Repeat 10 times and switch legs.

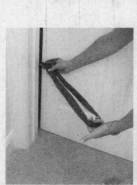

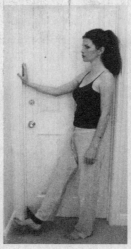

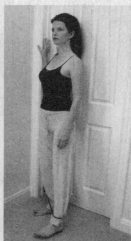

Figure 1	Figure 2	Figure 3

Thigh Toner

Buttocks Toner. Lie on your stomach and place your right ankle through the elastic band wedged in the door. Keep your pelvis and thigh muscles pushed hard into the floor as you bend the right knee and slowly pull the band up toward your buttocks with the right ankle. Do 10 repetitions and switch legs.

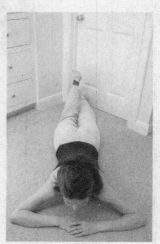

Buttocks Toner

PUTTING IT ALL TOGETHER

Most people find it best to do their stretching and strengthening routines at the same time or times each day so that it becomes a welcome and convenient ritual. Finding an efficient order of daily exercise, grouped by body position (e.g., standing first, lying face up and then face down) and stretching needs, will help. Here is an example of one routine that you might want to use exactly as is, cut back to fit your current fitness level, or build upon to create your own personalized workout routine.

Standing warm-up. Back leg stretch, hamstring stretch, quadriceps stretch, shoulder stretch, triceps stretch, biceps/chest stretch, elbow-wrist stretch, neck and shoulder stretch, chest stretch.

Floor workout. Abdominal crunch (lie on back), abdominal side toning, hip and inner thigh stretch, low back stretch, upper-body floor stretch (flip over, stomach on floor), extremity and torso strengthener, cat stretch, prayer stretch.

Stand-up strap routine. Biceps toner, triceps toner, shoulder and upper back toner, inner thigh toner, outer thigh toner, buttocks toner.

Let's Get Physical

The scientific evidence is convincing: physical fitness leads to brain fitness. Learning and getting in the habit of a repertoire of aerobic, toning, stretching, and muscle strengthening techniques will make everyone feel better, look more youthful, and, most of all, help to protect our minds and bodies from the effects of aging.

Physical Fitness Jump-Start

- Modify your routine of stretching and strengthening to individualize your Memory Prescription.
- Don't buy into the "no pain, no gain" myth.
- Try out several forms of aerobic workout to choose one that meets your needs and fits in with your lifestyle.
- Choose sports and activities that you enjoy because you are more likely to continue them in the long run.
- Consider augmenting your program with a fitness toy such as a treadmill, weight machine, or elastic band.
- Protect your back by strengthening your abdominal muscles and stretching your lower body.
- Choose sports and physical activities with low risk for head trauma. Wear helmets when riding bikes or doing sports.
- Check with your physician when getting started, especially if you have a physical illness that an exercise program could affect.

Chapter Ten:

Drugs and Supplements—Myths, Truths, and Consequences

You can tell if a man is healthy by what he takes two at a time —
stairs or pills.
— MILTON BERLE

Modern medicine plays a large role in the extended longevity so many people enjoy in today's "age revolution." Drugs and supplements have not only extended the average life expectancy, they have also improved our quality of life, allowing us to live longer *and* better.

As our knowledge of existing compounds grows at an escalating pace, so does the arrival of new medicines and formulas—some approved and understood by the medical community, and many that are not. We consumers are bombarded with information, misinformation, and myths about miracle cures for everything from cold sores to osteoporosis. Many of us tend to get distracted by the latest "grapefruit-soup-diet-formula that dissolves away fat cells while we sleep," or some "mega-libido-garlic-youth-capsule" claiming to perk up our sex lives until age 110. However, as a rule, if it sounds too good to be true, it probably is.

After each new drug or vaccine breakthrough in the fight against Alzheimer's disease, I receive a flurry of phone calls from folks pursuing that new panacea that will guarantee them protection from a dreaded mental decline or possibly cure their loved one of advancing dementia. Oftentimes people do improve with new medicines, even dramatically so. However, everybody responds to formulas differently, and it is important to maintain realistic expectations when trying new medications. In this chapter, we'll try to separate the science from the hype where medicines and supplements are concerned. We will take a look at many new and not-so-new medicines for protecting or even improving our brains and overall quality longevity.

The 14-Day Memory Prescription includes a basic, daily supplement regimen of omega-3 capsules, multivitamins, and antioxidant vitamins C and E. Many people, however, are interested in taking additional supplements, and I advise they first weigh the benefits versus the risks of not just the compound itself, but also the way in which it may react with other formulas they are currently taking. The best way I know to gather this information quickly is to discuss it with your doctor.

Follow Doctor's Orders

Chronic physical illnesses like diabetes or high blood pressure become more prevalent with age. The early symptoms are often subtle but, if left untreated, these kinds of common conditions can lead to impaired memory ability and diminished brain fitness. Along with effective medicines, the Memory Prescription's healthy diet, stress reduction techniques, and physical conditioning regimen will help prevent these illnesses or help people to control them.

DRUGS FOR HYPERTENSION

If you're over 65, then chances are greater than 50:50 that you have high blood pressure. Recent studies indicate that people with untreated, chronic high blood pressure during their forties and fifties suffer increased cognitive decline later in life. Many experts believe chronic hypertension affects memory because it thickens and stiffens blood vessels. Under high pressure, these stiffened blood vessels can rupture, and may cause cerebrovascular disease involving blood leakage into the brain tissue and eventual stroke. A stroke is often defined as the death of brain cells, resulting in a loss of physical or mental function, or both.

The good news is that hypertension is easily detected with a blood pressure cuff and stethoscope at your doctor's office or even using home devices, and it's effectively treated with a variety of antihypertensive medicines. However, these drugs are only recommended for people *with* hypertension. No evidence has ever supported their use as a treatment to maintain brain health in people with normal blood pressure. The most effective intervention for hypertension usually involves both medicine and lifestyle change. Quitting smoking and limiting excessive alcohol and food consumption can control blood pressure. Regular exercise, a low-salt diet, and avoidance of other high-risk activities all lower blood pressure.

CHOLESTEROL-LOWERING STATINS

Another potentially dangerous effect of aging is that our blood levels of cholesterol tend to rise. This waxy, soft substance has many functions in the body, forming cell membranes and hormones like estrogen or cortisol. Excess cholesterol, though, especially the "bad" LDL form, contributes to a damaging buildup of plaque in arteries throughout the body. In the brain, the plaque buildup impairs circulation and contributes to strokes that diminish memory ability.

Though our genetic inheritance partly determines our individual risk for high cholesterol as we age, lifestyle choices are a big factor. What you eat, whether or not you exercise, and your level of stress all play a role.

If you can't control your cholesterol with lifestyle changes, a group of drugs known as statins are what the doctor will usually order. Already an estimated 15 million Americans take these drugs, and new federal health guidelines recommend that 21 million more should use statins to prevent heart disease. Statin drugs save lives every year. If someone has a high cholesterol level, a statin drug will reduce their risk of death from heart attack by 30 to 40 percent. The drugs are so effective that some people use them to cheat on their low-fat diets. I know a baby boomer or two who have chosen to take a statin drug every day rather than give up their favorite steak house or French restaurant. Your doctor should be involved in such a decision—perhaps discuss it over dinner at that nice French restaurant . . .

Scientists recently observed that statin drugs not only lower fat levels in the blood, but they may also help prevent age-related memory decline and even lower risk for Alzheimer's disease. After a review of more than 60,000 hospital records, Dr. Benjamin Wolozin and Dr. George Siegel and their colleagues at Loyola University found that the rate of Alzheimer's disease in patients taking cholesterol-lowering statins, including lovastatin (Mevacor) and pravastatin (Pravachol), was nearly 75 percent lower when compared to the entire population, or to patients taking other medicines for different conditions such as hypertension or cardiovascular disease. Other statins that have been associated with a lower Alzheimer's risk include atorvastatin (Lipitor), fluvastatin (Lescol), and simvastatin (Zocor).

Statins work by blocking the liver's production of an enzyme necessary for cholesterol synthesis. Some experts speculate that the drugs protect the brain either through lowering cholesterol or through an anti-inflammatory effect, but there may be other reasons. Statins heighten levels of nitric oxide, a substance that helps keep blood vessel walls flexible enough for ample blood flow, and these healthier blood vessels may lower the risk of stroke. Other research linking cholesterol metabolism to the deposition of the amyloid plaques found in the Alzheimer's brain suggests that cholesterol-lowering drugs may interfere with this deadly protein deposition.

Although a recent double-blind test comparing the drug pravastatin against a placebo showed no benefit for people once they develop Alzheimer's disease, it is still possible that statins are effective in *preventing* the disease. Because we don't yet have results from prevention trials and statins do occasionally cause side effects—even, rarely, *causing* memory loss—most experts do not yet recommend statins as drugs to maintain brain health and stave off future memory loss.

ANTI-INFLAMMATORY DRUGS

Epidemiological studies have observed that using anti-inflammatory drugs, particularly a group known as nonsteroidal anti-inflammatory drugs (NSAIDs), may reduce the risk of getting Alzheimer's disease by as much as 60 percent if people took them for at least two years. These drugs are generally used to treat minor injuries and arthritis. Examples include aspirin, ibuprofen (Motrin, Advil, Nuprin), piroxicam (Feldene), naproxyn (Aleve), and indomethacin (Indocin).

Some scientists have theorized that the drugs' brain effects come from their action on inflammation, the body's natural defense mechanism against any outside intruder like bacteria or foreign objects, whether it's a splinter or a bullet. When pathologists examine the Alzheimer amyloid plaques under the microscope, they see a central core consisting of insoluble amyloid protein surrounded by an outer rim indicating an inflammatory reaction. This presumed inflammatory attack to rid the brain of amyloid protein causes cell death and memory loss.

Our research at UCLA points to another explanation. When Dr. Jorge Barrio and our other collaborators mixed anti-inflammatory drugs with Alzheimer plaques, the drugs literally dissolved the plaques away. Our conclusion was that some of these drugs might prevent Alzheimer's not necessarily because they stop brain inflammation, but instead from their ability to prevent the toxic amyloid protein from aggregating and building up in the brain.

More research is needed to get definitive answers as to how effective these medicines are and exactly how they may exert that effect. I recently commented to a friend that he seemed to be in particularly good physical and mental health. He had managed to avoid the typical midriff bulge of many baby boomers, and he was always witty and quick during conversation. He immediately gave me a discourse on his program of five-mile weekend runs, lunch-hour tennis dates, and so on. He smiled and held up a pill bottle saying, "Thank God for my anti-inflammatory drugs." Without them, he had too much pain and stiffness to keep up with his fitness program.

Sure, his anti-inflammatory drugs are keeping his joints in shape so he can maintain his high level of physical activity. They may even be protecting his brain cells from damaging inflammation. But there is another possible explanation to consider: his regular, long-term physical aerobic conditioning was also protecting his brain cells and keeping them fit, just as it was maintaining his cardiac fitness (see Chapter 9).

Although anti-inflammatory drugs do not appear to protect the brain once people develop full-blown dementia or Alzheimer's disease, research is under way to conclusively determine if they work as preventive treatments for people with only mild memory complaints. One recent investigation found that only a half-tablet of daily aspirin was sufficient to demonstrate an association with better cognition.

Anti-inflammatory drugs may have side effects for some people, including elevated blood pressure, kidney problems, and stomach bleeding, but newer drugs like Vioxx, Celebrex, and Bextra, known as cox-II inhibitors (they inhibit only one of the enzymes—cyclooxygenase II), have lower rates of these unwanted effects. Some studies, however, suggest that they may not be as effective brain protectors as the older drugs, like Motrin or Aleve. Because of these potential side effects and the lack of direct evidence for their protective effects, most experts would not yet recommend the use of anti-inflammatory drugs as preventive treatments for brain aging or Alzheimer's disease.

ANTIDEPRESSANTS

We all get sad and blue from time to time. For about 15 percent of the population, that sadness becomes so profound that they require medical attention at some point in their life. Antidepressant drugs are safe and effective for such clinical depressions.

When people get depressed, their negative thoughts distract them and diminish their ability to concentrate, especially as they age. When depressed middle-aged and older people often emphasize concentration difficulties, and they complain about memory slips. A form of depression often seen in older people has been labeled "pseudodementia" because it so closely resembles a dementia or Alzheimer's disease. A person who is overwhelmed by sadness and despair may have trouble trying to learn, and remembering new information is the last thing on their minds. Their sleep patterns are also disturbed, further aggravating memory abilities. It is known that episodes of repeated and severe depression can lead to abnormal secretion of stress hormones, and this can further worsen memory problems (Chapter 8).

Until recently, a stumbling block in treating older depressed people has been that originally available antidepressants like amitriptyline (Elavil) or imipramine (Tofranil) worsened memory loss. In fact, they worsened the brain messenger or neurotransmitter system that goes awry in Alzheimer's disease, the cholinergic system. Today, we have newer antidepressants, such as fluoxetine (Prozac), sertraline (Zoloft), or paroxetine (Paxil), to mention a few, that have much better side-effect profiles and work effectively to improve mood.

Medicine is only part of the answer for many depressions—talking to a professional may be preferred in many situations and often augments the antidepressant effect. Recent studies have found that in some older adults, combined symptoms of depression and memory loss may improve with antidepressant medication. However, such conditions may precede a more chronic, cognitive decline. For people who are *not* depressed, antidepressant medicines are *not* recommended as treatments to improve brain fitness and stave off future memory loss.

MEDICINES FOR OTHER ILLNESSES

My routine approach to evaluating a person's memory complaints includes a review of several medical conditions that can affect their brain function. Most medical conditions can be ruled out as the cause following a simple physical examination and screening laboratory tests, but for some patients, the antidementia drug of choice turns out to be a thyroid supplement or a medicine to control diabetes. Any acute illness that attacks our bodies can also overwhelm our brain capacity. Patients of any age have experienced temporary confusion and word-finding difficulties during flu or pneumonia. The take-home message is to follow the doctor's orders and take physical illnesses seriously in order to protect brain fitness and prevent future memory loss.

If a Little Medicine Is Good, Then Isn't a Lot Better?

So now you may have your cholesterol meds, your pills for blood pressure, and possibly those anti-inflammatory drugs. You may well want to get a pillbox to help you keep track of the various medications you are taking. If this is your scenario, don't panic—you are not alone. The average older adult takes more than half a dozen prescription medicines at any one time, but the more medicines we take, the greater the possibility for negative drug interactions.

I always ask new patients to bring in all their medications on the first visit. Sometimes a patient will arrive at my office with shopping bags filled with prescription bottles. Often merely eliminating unnecessary medicines and/or reducing their dosage levels will improve the patient's memory symptoms without further intervention.

Aging causes our brain receptors to become more sensitive to the effects of drugs, increasing the possibility of side effects at much lower doses. Also, our bodies become less efficient in breaking down and eliminating medicines, so over time we may accumulate higher blood levels of drugs. This can lead to new or increased side effects, as well as interactions with other drugs that we hadn't experienced in the past. Due to these changes in our bodies, doctors caring for older people often prescribe drugs in low doses initially and slowly increase them as needed to minimize any potential adverse reactions.

Many medications have anticholinergic side effects, meaning they oppose the actions of the drugs prescribed for memory loss, thereby worsening memory. Also, I am often concerned about the drugs prescribed for anxiety—such as Xanax, Valium, or Librium—which are frequently overused and can cause sedation and memory impairment. Even drugs used to regulate heart rate or treat high blood pressure can make blood vessels less taut and decrease the heart's ability to pump blood. Since our vascular tone diminishes anyway as we age, medicines that aggravate this problem can lead to falls, head trauma, and other complications that threaten brain fitness, and they should be taken with care.

With the advent of new drugs to treat cancer, a new form of mental side effect has emerged, often referred to as "chemo brain." Doctors initially ignored these memory complaints, attributing them to indirect expressions of anxiety or depression, but such cognitive deficits are now recognized as real side effects of cancer treatments. Although usually mild in severity, they reportedly affect up to 40 percent of patients taking these drugs. Doctors are puzzled about the cause of chemo brain since most of the drugs used to treat cancer do not actually cross the blood-brain barrier, the protective membrane that filters substances circulating between the bloodstream and the brain. But the memory deficits are real and could result from indirect effects of the drugs on natural chemicals in the body. Treatments for the condition are still in their infancy, but scientists are considering stimulants, as well as drugs used to treat Alzheimer's disease.

If you are concerned that medication may be affecting your memory, consult your physician about whether you truly need a particular drug, and be sure the doctor is aware of all the medicines you currently take. This is especially important if you are under the care of more than one physician.

Should Everyone Take Anti-Alzheimer's Drugs?

While recently arguing the case for the use of PET scans to help doctors make an early and more effective diagnosis of Alzheimer's disease, I noted that even those who still resisted the costs of investing in this new imaging technology had to agree that the PET scans improved diagnostic accuracy.

However, they argued that since the available anti-Alzheimer's drugs are relatively safe, why not skip the diagnosis and just give the drugs to everyone with memory complaints?

Although prescribing the same treatment to everyone, regardless of their actual diagnosis, may not be the most effective approach, there is the possibility that some anti-Alzheimer's drugs may soon be available for people with only mild cognitive impairment, a condition of memory loss that is not considered a disease state, but instead indicates a risk of about 10 percent annually for developing dementia. Several of these available medicines are currently being tested to see if they can delay the onset of dementia. I believe it is likely that within the next few years several anti-Alzheimer's medicines will be approved for actual prevention of the disease.

CHOLINESTERASE INHIBITORS AS BRAIN BOOSTERS?

New studies support the idea that treating early brain-aging symptoms with cholinergic drugs—medicines currently used to treat Alzheimer's disease—may actually interfere with the deposition of amyloids, the insoluble proteins that have accumulated in the brains of people with the disease. Because this cholinergic brain-messenger system appears to decline with normal aging, it is possible that taking a cholinesterase inhibitor drug as a brain booster or smart drug could benefit many people experiencing "senior moments" or "middle-age pauses."

Cholinergic drugs enhance the body's level of acetylcholine, the chemical neurotransmitter that facilitates passage of nerve impulses across brain synapses. The brains of Alzheimer's patients have a deficiency of acetylcholine, which can result from either impaired production or excess breakdown by enzymes called cholinesterases, and our currently approved treatments inhibit these enzymes, so they are called "cholinesterase inhibitors."

Tacrine (Cognex) was the first of these medicines to be approved, but it is now rarely used due to the extent of its side effects. The newer compounds have fewer side effects and include donepezil (Aricept, approved by the FDA in November 1996), rivastigmine (Exelon, approved in April 2000), and galantamine (Reminyl, approved May 2001). These drugs not only improve memory and thinking, but they can also reduce agitation and depression. Recent research shows that they benefit patients with different forms of dementia, including dementia with Lewy bodies, vascular dementia, and even mixed dementias. Some experts have reported poor results in patients with frontotemporal dementia, although systematic studies have not proven this observation. Aricept, Exelon, and Reminyl are all currently being tested to determine whether they can delay the onset of dementia in people with mild cognitive impairment.

NMDA RECEPTOR ANTAGONIST

Memantine (Namenda), a drug used for decades in Europe, was recently approved for treatment of dementia in the United States. Rather than influencing the cholinergic transmitter system, memantine works on the brain's NMDA receptors by blocking the brain chemical glutamate, which overstimulates these receptors, allowing too much calcium to enter cells, leading to cell destruction. When taken in doses of 20 milligrams daily, Namenda benefits patients with moderate to severe Alzheimer's disease, but many clinicians find that it is effective in milder forms of memory loss as well.

Another encouraging observation of memantine is the additional benefit it brings to many patients already taking a cholinesterase inhibitor drug. A recent study found that dementia patients already taking the cholinesterase inhibitor drug Aricept for an average of six months showed additional benefit and slower memory decline when they added Namenda to their treatment regimen, compared with those who remained on the Aricept without added Namenda. Encouraged by the drug's different mechanism of action, more studies are planned to determine whether Namenda may be useful to treat mild age-related memory loss and to possibly prevent future cognitive decline.

OTHER MEMORY-ENHANCING DRUGS

A variety of other memory-enhancing drugs have been considered for the treatment of full-blown dementia, as well as mild age-related memory impairment. Such drugs as physostigmine and hydergine generated excitement in previous years, but mixed results from studies have dampened enthusiasm for their memory-enhancing effects. Ampakines and clioquiniline are currently under study as possible treatments for various degrees of cognitive deficit. Appendix 5 provides additional information on such memory enhancing drugs.

Hormones for Brain Power

Scientists have shown considerable interest in understanding how these natural chemical communicators might improve memory performance. The fact that they are natural makes them attractive to the public as brain, muscle, and libido boosters. But natural may not mean safe and, to date, studies have not convinced all experts that their potential benefits outweigh their risks.

DHEA (DEHYDROEPIANDROSTERONE)

Secreted by the body's adrenal gland, DHEA is a building block for our sex hormones, estrogen and testosterone. Side effects include an increased risk for prostate cancer, facial hair growth, scalp balding, and acne. Athletes take DHEA to build strength and bulk before big events despite its recent ban by organizations like the National Football League and International Olympic Committee. The FDA banned its over-the-counter sale back in 1985 when it was marketed for weight loss, but in 1994 the ruling was reversed. Its potential for protecting brain cells suggested promise for treating dementia and memory loss, but systematic studies have not panned out.

GROWTH HORMONE STIMULANTS

Pick up any men's magazine or browse the Internet on how to build muscle mass and trim fat, and you'll learn about natural products thought to trigger the release of chemical messengers. Companies marketing "hormone releaser" pills say their products are a cheaper, needle-free alternative to more traditional human growth hormone treatments. The active ingredient is often arginine or another amino acid that signals the pituitary gland to release or secrete growth hormone. But taking arginine has no such effect, and you can get the same dose of amino acids by eating a six-ounce steak, which tastes much better. For now, muscle-building athletes and older men who tend to take them should be cautious because of the potential side effects and the minimal evidence thus far of any benefit.

ESTROGEN

In recent years, scientists have taken increasing interest in the effects of estrogen and other hormones on mood and memory in older adults. The Women's Health Initiative Memory Study recently found that women age 65 and older taking a particular estrogen plus progestin hormone therapy had twice the rate of developing dementia, including Alzheimer's disease, compared with women who did not take the medication. The study also found that the combination therapy did not protect the women against the development of mild cognitive impairment, a different form of cognitive decline that is less severe than dementia. Short-term hormone therapy in younger women to relieve some symptoms of menopause has been approved by the U.S. Food and Drug Administration, but there is little known about the long-term effects. Women of any age should consult with their doctor about their individual needs, risks, and benefits.

TESTOSTERONE

An estimated 600,000 men in the United States use some form of prescription testosterone each year to augment their levels in an attempt to cure their memory complaints, fatigue, low sex drive, and shrinking muscle mass. The expected age-related testosterone dips are subtle and occur gradually over decades, and only about one out of five men 65 and older end up with an abnormally low testosterone level. Many proponents argue that we ought to treat general malaise, low energy, and diminished libido with testosterone, noting that if it improves quality of life, why not? However, overuse can have a down side. Testosterone stimulates prostate cancer growth, and the majority of older men have inactive cancer cells in their prostates which excess testosterone use could awaken. Initial studies indicate that men with low levels do experience improvements in mood and memory following testosterone administration, but systematic study is still needed to prove a true benefit for memory performance and brain health.

Dietary Supplements

Dietary supplements have become a popular form of alternative therapy throughout the world. In the United States, a 1997 survey reported that more than 12 percent of adults had used some kind of herbal supplement in the previous year, compared with less than 3 percent seven years earlier. Also, as we get older, we may be more inclined to use supplements. Another recent survey indicated that more than 40 percent of men and 50 percent of women age 60 and older reported using at least one supplement.

Most herbal remedies in the United States are considered dietary supplements, so they are not regulated as medicines. In 1994, the Dietary Supplement Health and Education Act set forth the only standards for manufacturers, who are responsible for the truthfulness of label claims. Manufacturers must have evidence that supports their claims, but the FDA provides no standard for that evidence, nor does it require they submit that evidence.

Consumers face several challenges when deciding whether or not to take these popular products. Even if an herbal remedy is effective, there is limited quality control from brand to brand, and there is no guarantee of effectiveness. Just because a dietary supplement is natural does not necessarily mean it is safe, and health risks may emerge from drug interactions or contaminants. Problems including excess bleeding, pain, insomnia, and even more serious drug interactions have been reported with various supplements. For example, ingesting ginkgo along with caffeine can lead to blood clots surrounding the brain (subdural hematomas), and ginkgo can affect insulin secretion, making it potentially dangerous for diabetics.

When deciding on which form or brand of supplement to take, consumers need accurate information about the level of evidence on both the supplement's safety and its effectiveness. A knowledgeable pharmacist or physician can often help. Other informative resources include the National Center for Complementary and Alternative Medicine (nccam.nih.gov) and the Natural Medicines Comprehensive Database (www.naturaldatabase.com). You can also contact my Web site at www.drgarysmall.com for further information. Dietary supplements are available in most vitamin, food, and drugstores nationwide.

ACETYL-L-CARNITINE

This nutrient helps the body metabolize fats, produce energy, and make the memory-promoting neurotransmitter acetylcholine. Acetyl-l-carnitine may also function as an antioxidant and cell-membrane stabilizer. University of California biochemist Dr. Bruce Ames has noted the potential memory benefits of combining acetyl-l-carnitine with the antioxidant lipoic acid. Daily dosages range from 1.5 to 4 grams in divided doses.

COENZYME Q$_{10}$

Because of its antioxidant properties, some people have used this supplement to treat age-related memory loss or to slow the progression of Alzheimer's disease, although systematic research is limited. Coenzyme Q_{10} can interact with medicines used to treat heart failure, diabetes, and kidney or liver problems. Typical doses range from 100 to 300 milligrams daily.

CREATINE

A new study from the University of Sydney in Australia found that taking 5 grams of this supplement each day improved memory ability and intellectual functioning in young adult volunteers compared to controls taking a placebo. Though encouraging, this represents just one study and creatine does have a potential down side. Long-term use may have a negative impact on glucose equilibrium in the body and the supplement can cause an unpleasant body odor.

CURCUMIN

Curcumin is the yellow spice found in curry powder, and it gives mustard its bright color. Laboratory studies have demonstrated its anti-inflammatory and antioxidant effects, which may protect brain cells. Curcumin is currently under study as a treatment for mild memory loss and dementia in doses ranging from 200 to 1,000 milligrams daily.

DIMETHYLAMINOETHANOL (DMAE)

Because of its effect on the brain's cholinergic messenger system involved in learning and recall, DMAE may benefit patients with age-related memory decline and Alzheimer's disease, though results of systematic studies are not available. DMAE is generally safe, but occasionally causes insomnia, confusion, or elevated blood pressure. Typical dosages range from 100 to 400 milligrams daily in divided doses.

DL-PHENYLALANINE

This combination of essential amino acids has been used to promote mental functioning, mood, and muscle relaxation. The compound serves as a building block for neurotransmitters known to support emotional well-being, memory, and learning, and may regulate the levels of endorphins, the body's own natural antidepressant. Some experts have also recommended the compound to assist with mild age-related memory complaints, though results of systematic studies are not available. Dosages prescribed are often in the 500 milligrams twice daily range.

GINKGO BILOBA

Ginkgo may improve cognitive function through brain circulation or antioxidant effects. It also boosts the absorption of glucose, the brain's main fuel source, and facilitates several brain messengers important to memory. Some but not all studies have demonstrated significant cognitive benefits. Because many of the studies have limitations in their methods, better-designed investigations are currently underway, including a large trial comparing ginkgo biloba to placebo in approximately 3,000 people age 75 or older. Ginkgo occasionally causes nausea, heartburn, headaches, dizziness, bleeding, or low blood pressure, though for most people it is relatively safe, especially if they have their doctor review their other medicines to ensure against potential drug interactions. People who decide to take ginkgo should use a high-quality preparation. The recommended daily dosage is 120 milligrams in divided doses.

HUPERZINE A

Huperzine acts to inhibit the cholinesterase enzyme, making the acetylcholine brain messenger more available to stimulate neurons. Although not all studies have been positive, several investigations have demonstrated huperzine benefits in patients with dementia, and initial experience in people with mild states of memory loss is promising. Doses range from 50 micrograms twice daily for milder memory loss to 500 micrograms twice daily for dementia.

LECITHIN

A major component of all living cells, lecithin is broken down in the body to active cholinergic compounds that have minimal but inconsistent memory benefits. Systematic studies do not support the use of lecithin in the treatment of patients with dementia or other cognitive impairments.

MELATONIN

The principal hormone secreted by the pineal gland, melatonin is a brain messenger with a structure similar to serotonin, the same brain messenger that requires augmenting in many depressions. Its antioxidant activity has led investigators to consider it as a treatment against Alzheimer's disease, but the limited data thus far do not yet support its use.

OMEGA-3 SUPPLEMENTS

For people who wish to ensure adequate brain protection from fish oils, use supplements that include such omega-3 fats as docosahexaenoic acid or DHA, which increases the acetylcholine memory-promoting neurotransmitter. Recent studies suggest that omega-3-rich supplements may help a person's mood as well as their memory. Omega-3 fats also minimize brain inflammation that can damage neurons and have an antioxidant effect that fights against free radicals that can further injure brain cells. The usual recommended dosage is 1,000 milligrams of an omega-3 supplement each day, the amount included in the Memory Prescription Diet. Also, these supplements usually contain fish oil and flaxseed oil, both of which are extremely sensitive to light and to air oxidation. Make sure that you purchase the supplements from a store that keeps them refrigerated and buy in small quantities.

PHOSPHATIDYLSERINE

Scientists have found that phosphatidylserine increases neurotransmitters that improve memory and concentration. Numerous studies have found that this supplement benefits memory and learning more than a placebo sugar pill in people with mild age-related memory complaints. Though encouraging in the short run, the studies have been relatively brief in duration, ranging from 6 to 12 weeks, raising the possibility that the benefit may not be long-term. Doctors who recommend phosphatidylserine suggest that people begin with 100 to 150 milligrams twice a day and after several months they drop the dose to only 50 milligrams twice a day for maintenance. No side effects have been reported.

VINPOCETINE

Vinpocetine has several effects that might improve memory performance and maintain brain fitness, including its ability to enhance circulation in the brain, as well as its antioxidant properties. Vinpocetine has been tested against placebo sugar pills in studies of patients with dementia and normal volunteers. Several but not all studies demonstrate significant memory benefits within a few days and for up to three months. Usual recommended daily dosages range from 10 to 80 milligrams in divided doses.

A Vitamin Each Day May Really Keep the Doctor Away

The Memory Prescription includes a multivitamin supplement not only to protect us against deficiencies but also to guard against oxidants and age related illness. Infection risks increase with age, and taking a single multiple vitamin capsule may bolster our immune function and protect us against infections.

It appears that a daily multivitamin may do more than just keep the doctor away. It may also keep our memory performance in top form. For example, daily β-carotene use is associated with better memory performance in older individuals. Volunteers taking thiamine, riboflavin, niacin, and folate supplements score better in abstract thinking tests. People with heightened blood levels of vitamin C score higher on tests of visual and spatial ability.

Because 20 percent of people age 60 and older, and 40 percent of those over age 80, lose some of their ability to absorb vitamin B_{12}, many experts advise older adults to take this B vitamin supplement, in addition to their daily multivitamin. The antioxidant B vitamin folate, or folic acid, protects us from developing strokes and heart disease. Some studies have shown that when Alzheimer's victims are treated with high doses of vitamin B_{12} or folate, their memory abilities improve.

People who eat well-balanced meals generally don't develop deficiencies, and most doctors recommend daily multiple vitamins to ensure that such deficiencies do not develop. We also should keep in mind the potential toxic effects of unnecessary vitamin megadoses. This may be a particular problem with fat-soluble vitamins such as vitamins A, D, E, and K, which get stored in our body fat and can hang around in our bodies for weeks, months, or longer. When a little bit is good, a lot isn't always better.

The Antioxidant Movement

In Chapter 7, we learned how free radicals that are everywhere in the environment work to wear down our brain cells and eventually destroy them if left unchecked. To help control this destructive oxidative process, we are wise to choose generously from the many colorful fruits and vegetables that can hold back these relentless attacks on our brain cells.

If you're like myself and many other memory fitness fanatics, you want some extra ammunition to use in the antioxidant wars. Rather than just relying on the natural antioxidants in our foods, a few selected supplements are an attractive add-on to a healthy brain regimen. The two major vitamin supplements used to combat those pesky free radicals are vitamins E and C.

People with low blood levels of these antioxidant vitamins have poorer memory abilities. Epidemiologists who've followed people in their communities while testing their memory and other cognitive performances report that those taking supplemental vitamin C and E tablets appear to have better memory abilities and less cognitive decline over time. One recent four-year study of people over age 65 found that not one of the subjects who regularly took the antioxidant vitamins C and E developed Alzheimer's disease.

Unfortunately, most studies of the effects of antioxidant vitamins on memory performance only record whether or not the participant was taking a supplement beyond just a daily multivitamin tablet, which generally contains about 30 units of vitamin E and 60 milligrams of vitamin C. The investigators have not determined the optimal vitamin supplement dosage for preventing Alzheimer's disease. Exactly how much your doctor might recommend for you is a matter of clinical judgment.

For healthy people who wish to take antioxidant supplements as part of their healthy brain diet, I recommend a daily dose of 400 to 800 units of vitamin E, and 500 to 1,000 milligrams of vitamin C. Increased bleeding and stomach upset can occur at higher doses of vitamin E, and some studies suggest that male smokers who take vitamin E supplements have higher mortality rates. However, for most people, antioxidant vitamins are extremely safe. These vitamins not only help protect our brains, but they also defend our bodies against some forms of cancer, diabetes, and Parkinson's disease, as well as increase our immune defenses against colds and viruses. If you have questions, consult your doctor before taking a supplement.

Keeping Your Brain Young with Drugs and Supplements

- Numerous physical illnesses can age your brain. Take them seriously—see your doctor sooner rather than later.
- Avoid using more medicines than you need. Talk with your doctor about any drugs you are taking that could influence memory ability.
- Remember that treating a depression with the right antidepressant drug often improves memory performance.
- Know about the potential benefits and risks of dietary supplements before deciding whether to take them.
- If you decide to use supplements, pick brands with good quality and safety records.
- Always inform your doctor about over-the-counter medicines and dietary supplements you are taking.

Chapter Eleven:

Renewing Your Prescription— A Lifetime of Quality Longevity

I don't want to achieve immortality through my work.
I want to achieve immortality through not dying.
—WOODY ALLEN

When you have completed the first two weeks of your program, you will probably have more confidence in just about all of your everyday memory tasks. You may feel sharper mentally and experience more energy, while others may be commenting that you appear more attentive and even look better, especially if you dropped a pound or two on the Memory Prescription Diet.

But now you may be wondering: "Can I keep up these new healthy habits beyond two weeks? Even with my newly improved memory skills, can I remember everything to do to keep up my program?" As one of my patients recently put it, "Doc, tell me how I can *renew* my Memory Prescription."

This chapter will help you stay on track by providing a basic framework to continue your Memory Prescription for the next two weeks, the two weeks after that, and the rest of your life. It will be easier than you think because you've already done the hardest work. You've followed the program just long enough for the new lifestyle habits to take hold and to make a difference in your life. Most people customize their program in the beginning, often without even realizing it, and I didn't design the Memory Prescription 14-Day Plan expecting you to follow every recommendation, 100 percent of the time.

The key to maintaining and building your program over the next several weeks, months, and years is to expand on some of the organizational skills I touched upon in Chapter 6, when you learned advanced memory training techniques. To show you how it works, I will use several examples from people of different ages and varied lifestyles: a 42-year-old "sandwich generation" caregiver, a 21-year-old college student, a 55-year-old executive, and a 69-year-old retired contractor. To organize your Memory Prescription renewal plan, I have included work sheets that will help you chart your progress until the new memory fitness habits simply become a way of life, a path to living better, longer.

Adding to Brain Efficiency with External Aids

Our brains are like computers in that each of us has a limited amount of memory capacity. No matter how well we learn mnemonic techniques (Chapters 3 and 6), there will always be too much information to retain in our memory stores. Even people with extraordinary ability for memorizing lists of trivia have limitations in their ability to store facts and figures. Many of the people who succeed in learning and recall skills, and in life in general, have learned to choose which information is useful to learn and which information is less important and might be glossed over. As you renew your prescription, allow yourself to utilize *external memory tools* or aids such as to-do lists and day planners, as well as the *internal memory tools* or mnemonic techniques you have been learning. Studies have found that using these kinds of external memory tools will enhance the effectiveness of your internal tools (e.g., *LOOK, SNAP, CONNECT*), even when you *don't* use an external tool at the time you recall the information. For example, the act of writing down items on a short list can sometimes fix those items into your memory, rendering it unnecessary to refer back to the list in order to recall the items.

Practicing *LOOK, SNAP, CONNECT* and other mnemonic techniques will provide you with greater brain efficiency—new information will be easier to learn and recall. External tools will give you an additional brain-efficiency punch. Here are some strategies that will help keep your memory abilities at peak performance and assist in renewing your prescription.

EFFECTIVE NOTES

Well-written summary notes condense the amount of material we have to re-member, and sometimes the simple act of writing things down helps facilitate recall. The more thought and effort we put into creating a note of something to remember, the more helpful it will be. Some college students have reported that simply rewriting their class notes more neatly the night after a lecture, is enough "study time" to secure the information into their memory stores.

MEMORY PLACES

To avoid the "disappearing keys act," put commonly misplaced items in the same "memory" place—a hook near the door in the kitchen for your car keys, the same briefcase pocket for your organizer, and that convenient desk drawer for the scissors and the pencils. Your office, home, and car can be more efficient if the storage areas and living spaces are organized with desig-nated memory places.

DAILY PLANNING LISTS

I developed this common technique for myself while I was training in medi-cine. The best way for me to keep track of my patient-care tasks was to make lists, and once I completed a task, I'd cross it off. I still use these daily lists, and after a few days, I transfer the remaining active items to a new list. If the list gets too long or complex, I place asterisks next to items that need more immediate attention.

WEEKLY OR MONTHLY PLANNING CALENDARS

A wall or desk calendar is a helpful way to keep track of regular or occasional events or meetings. Many families find it helpful to display one prominently in the kitchen or family room to remind them of upcoming family or school events.

DATE BOOKS, ELECTRONIC HAND-HELD ORGANIZERS

Pocket date books can help us keep track of the details in our lives, and lately electronic pocket gadgets have replaced date books because of their many programs, including calendars, phone books, and to-do lists, as well as Internet access. You can download the information onto your desktop computer so you can print it out, and should you lose your hand-held organizer, you won't lose all the information you've entered into it.

POST-ITS

Many people prefer Post-its or stick-on reminder notes as external memory aids. If you haven't tried them, you might consider using them to augment your other strategies. They are a good quick fix as a reminder, but try not to overuse them. A risk in using stick-on notes is that sometimes they "un-stick," though a new, especially sticky version is now available.

MEMORY HABITS

We begin learning memory habits from the time we are small children. We brush our teeth morning and night, and look both ways before crossing the street. We take vitamins after breakfast. As we get older, we continue to form new memory habits. If your dentist notes your chronic flossing deficit, you might create a new memory habit by placing the floss next to the toothpaste. If someone gives you a package you don't want to forget, you might place your car keys with it on the table—you won't get too far without taking the package when you leave. Daily pillbox organizers, alarm clocks, watches, and other tools are available to augment memory habits.

DAILY ROUTINES

Almost everyone functions better with a certain amount of structure in their lives. After two weeks on your program, some of your new routines may be starting to come naturally. If we build a general routine into our daily schedule, we will have more time to focus on work, leisure, and others things we want to learn.

PICK AND CHOOSE YOUR MEMORY AIDS

Creating too many lists, placing Post-its all over your dashboard, and lugging around a date book so jam-packed that you can't make out who you are lunching with won't necessarily be useful or effective in augmenting your memory abilities. Just as taking random, copious notes that are never read tends to be a waste of energy. On the other hand, succinct lists, notes, and reminders can be extremely helpful memory tools, and I sometimes keep mine for years. Picking and choosing the right memory tool can be as important as picking and choosing the information you wish to remember.

Building Tools to Renew Your Prescription

An effective way to renew your prescription is to create worksheets that serve as external memory tools that track your progress in each of the Big 4 areas of your program. The following worksheets will help you individualize your plan so you can emphasize areas that need additional work. You can use these as templates to design your own worksheets and make copies for each week ahead. To further guide you on using the worksheets, refer to the results of your questionnaire assessments after you completed the 14-Day Plan (Chapter 4). You might also want to glance at the information in each of the chapters focusing on the Big 4:

- **Stress Reduction—Chapter 8**
- **Diet—Chapter 7**

- **Mental Activity—Chapters 5 (mental aerobics) and 6 (memory training)**
- **Physical Conditioning—Chapter 9**

Over time, you will find that you no longer need the worksheets, since your healthy brain and body lifestyle habits will become ingrained in your long-term memory stores.

STRESS REDUCTION WORKSHEET

TASK	Mon.	Tues.	Wed.	Thurs.	Fri.	Sat.	Sun.
Sleep							
Multitasking							
Stress-release exercises							
Work/leisure ratio							
Physical exercise							
Relaxation breaks							

STRESS REDUCTION WORKSHEET GUIDE

1. *Sleep*: Record the number of hours in a 24-hour period. The average person needs 7 to 8 hours, but fewer with age. Insomniacs see Chapter 8.

2. *Multitasking*: Make a check each time you catch yourself.

3. *Stress-release exercises*: These may include any of those you learned in Chapters 3 or 8. Record the total amount of time spent.

4. *Work/leisure ratio*: Divide work hours by leisure hours. Strive to increase or decrease the ratio, depending on your needs.

5. *Physical exercise*: To reduce stress, build up your aerobic conditioning. Record the amount of time exercising each day. Cross reference with physical conditioning worksheet.

6. *Relaxation breaks*: Record the amount of time you spend doing nothing and chilling out.

7. *Blank rows*: Use these to record the amount of time you spend on other stress-release approaches of your choice. Record the duration of each session and note the type of activity (e.g., yoga, tai chi, meditation, self-hypnosis, biofeedback, massage, acupuncture, anger management, psychotherapy, etc.).

8. Don't get stressed out—you don't have to do everything on this worksheet. Choose what works for you and ignore the rest.

MEMORY PRESCRIPTION DIET WORKSHEET

TASK	Mon.	Tues.	Wed.	Thurs.	Fri.	Sat.	Sun.
Total calories							
Water							
Omega-3 fats							
Omega-6 fats							
Antioxidant foods							
Low glycemic index carbs							
High glycemic index carbs							
Caffeine							
Alcohol							

MEMORY PRESCRIPTION DIET WORKSHEET GUIDE

1. *Total calories*: If weight loss or weight gain is an issue for you, keep track of your daily calories to help you meet your goals.

2. *Water*: Shoot for eight glasses each day to stay hydrated and control weight.

3. *Fats*: Make sure you get enough omega-3 fatty acids in your diet. Emphasize fish, olive oil, and green leafy sources. You can also continue taking a 1,000 milligram omega-3 supplement for insurance. Try to limit animal fats, butter, mayonnaise, processed foods, fried foods, and vegetable oils.

4. *Antioxidants*: Record the approximate number of daily ORAC units and aim for at least 3,500 units (see chart on page 171 for ORAC ratings of different foods).

5. *Carbohydrates*: Emphasize natural foods (low glycemic index) and avoid those tempting desserts and foods with refined sugar (high glycemic index). (See ratings on page 175.)

6. *Caffeine*: Record daily number of cups of coffee or other sources of caffeine.

7. *Alcohol*: All things in moderation, and moderation in all things, especially alcoholic ones.

8. *Blank rows*: Use these to record progress on any special dietary goals (low salt, cholesterol control, vegetarian, etc.).

9. Limit your intake of high-mercury-containing fish like swordfish, shark, red snapper, and orange roughy.

10. Be sure to take your daily supplements. Refer to Chapter 10 for more information.

11. Try to eat at least five meals per day: breakfast, mid-morning snack, lunch, afternoon snack, and dinner.

MENTAL ACTIVITY WORKSHEET

TASK	Mon.	Tues.	Wed.	Thurs.	Fri.	Sat.	Sun.
Left-brain aerobics							
Right-brain aerobics							
Crosswords							
LOOK, SNAP, CONNECT							
Names and faces							
Story method							
Organization methods							
Peg method							

MENTAL ACTIVITY WORKSHEET GUIDE

1. *Left-brain aerobics*: Record the time you spend on mental activities that stimulate your left brain (e.g., logic, language, reading, math).

2. *Right brain aerobics*: Record time spent on activities that stimulate your right brain (e.g., artistic/musical tasks, visual/spatial, humor).

3. *Crosswords*: Try the daily newspapers—editors increase difficulty levels over the week (Monday is the easiest). Record daily times.

4. *LOOK, SNAP, CONNECT*: This is your foundation for most of your memory techniques. Record time each day you practice until you have it down.

5. *Names and faces*: Note how well you do with new people.

6. *Story method*: Apply to errands and other lists. Record how often you use it and how well you do.

7. *Organization methods*: Use categories, chunking, calendars, lists, memory places, and other organizational techniques.

8. *Peg method*: This optional method for card sharks and other memory masters requires practice before you can use it effectively. Record your progress if you dare to pursue it.

9. *Blank rows*: Memory training and mental aerobics can take many forms, including dancing, board games, learning a language, reading, etc.

10. If your job is mentally taxing, you may wish to play down or even avoid a daily mental aerobic workout.

11. Keep building your level over time. Make it challenging but not too tough, so you train but do not strain your brain.

PHYSICAL CONDITIONING WORKSHEET

TASK	Mon.	Tues.	Wed.	Thurs.	Fri.	Sat.	Sun.
Walking							
Jogging							
Cycling							
Swimming							
Stretching							
Muscle toning							

PHYSICAL CONDITIONING WORKSHEET GUIDE

1. *Physical aerobic conditioning*: Record the time you spend on activities that build your aerobic stamina, such as walking, jogging, swimming, racquet sports, etc.

2. *Stretching*: Record the amount of time spent and note the type of stretching. You may want to use additional rows for more complicated stretching routines.

3. *Muscle toning*: Record the amount of time spent and note the type of muscle toning exercise.

4. *Blank rows*: Use these rows to record your progress on other physical conditioning activities or to further detail those listed above.

5. Make sure that you try out several forms of aerobic workout so you can choose one that meets your needs and fits in with your lifestyle. You'll be more likely to stick with sports and activities that you enjoy.

6. Consider augmenting your program with a fitness toy such as a treadmill, weight machine, or inexpensive elastic band.

7. Check with your physician when getting started, especially if you have a physical illness that an exercise program could affect.

Use Visuals to Chart Your Progress

If you have a particular area that requires extra work, whether it's stress reduction, weight loss, or memory training, pick a daily or weekly target and chart your progress on a graph. That will allow you to see your improvement, as well as your skids backward. Observing the slides should help motivate you to shoot for your target.

The following is an example of one such graph for Jim B., who was trying to build up his aerobic conditioning, but an injury slowed him down. On Monday, Jim started building his jogging time rapidly over just a few days, perhaps too rapidly because he twisted his ankle on Thursday and had to cut the workout short. On the following day, he wisely switched to swimming, which allowed him to heal his ankle yet still continue to build his aerobic conditioning.

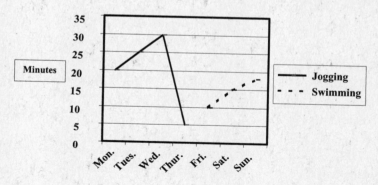

Eventually, Jim also got into a regular stretching routine that protected his legs and ankles from injury and allowed him to get back to his aerobic workout of choice—jogging.

Renewing Your Prescription: How It's Done

To get a better idea of how you, too, can renew your prescription, let's look at examples of several individuals from different walks of life. Each needed to emphasize different aspects of the Big 4 to maintain optimum memory fitness and brain health.

THE 42-YEAR-OLD
"SANDWICH GENERATION" CAREGIVER

Rose Z. had quite a lot on her plate even before her mother's hip surgery. Besides her part-time job, she had to drive her 12-year-old son to basketball practice after school twice a week, and her 9-year-old daughter to ballet lessons on Thursdays. The carpool helped, but Rose had to drive that two days a week as well. After her mother's surgery, Rose's hectic schedule got thrown off completely. On top of her job, all the other driving and the worry about her mother's health, Rose had to make time to visit her mother in the rehab facility, take mom to the doctors, and spend what seemed like hours listening to her complaints over the telephone.

The multitasking and stress began to erode Rose's usual precise memory skills. She started rushing out of the house without her car keys or her purse. She would forget to return client calls at work and actually missed a parent-teacher conference for the first time. She decided that she had to tackle this problem when she got a call from her tearful daughter who wanted to know when her mom was coming to pick her up from ballet—all the other kids were gone already.

The Memory Prescription had the formula that worked for Rose. She decided to start the 14-Day Plan during winter vacation when she had a break from her regular carpooling insanity. Plus, her sister came to visit, relieving her of some of the parent-care burden. With the 14-Day Plan, Rose felt great and experienced much less stress. Her old memory skills returned after the initial two weeks. When she renewed her Prescription, she emphasized the organizational techniques in the program. Rose bought herself a handheld organizer and got a large calendar for the kitchen to ensure that she would never again forget a carpool assignment or school event. Because the Memory Prescription's stress reduction exercises were so helpful initially, she wanted to augment that aspect of her program over time. Though she didn't have time to get to a yoga studio, she picked up a videotape on yoga and began her own stress-reduction exercise program at home.

THE 21-YEAR-OLD COLLEGE STUDENT

Andrea T. was a junior at an ivy-league college. Though she had gotten straight As in high school, she found herself struggling to keep up with her brainy college classmates, barely able to eke out a B+ average. Just before returning for her senior year, Andrea completed the 14-Day Plan—her mother's enthusiasm for the program caught her attention and she thought she might be able to lose the five pounds that she had gained last semester—that advanced pre-med lab elective really stressed her out. She was worried about the start of her senior year because she had the additional burden of preparing for her medical school admissions test. She wanted to protect herself from getting too stressed out that coming year.

In renewing her Prescription, Andrea was not thinking so much about improving her memory ability but more about improving her grades and doing well on her pre-med exams. She also wanted to lose a few more pounds and keep the weight off. Andrea's challenge was to figure out how to fit her new Memory Prescription habits into a busy academic year.

When she returned to school, Andrea completely dropped any mental aerobic workout—she was getting plenty in her daily studies and courses. For the first few weeks, she continued to practice *LOOK, SNAP, CONNECT*—it really streamlined her studying in classes with lots of material that required memorization. In fact, her studying was so much more efficient that she now had time for a daily jog. The additional exercise reduced her level of stress, gave her more confidence, and actually seemed to curb her appetite so she was able to cut her portions and keep her weight down. When her two roommates saw how great she looked after summer vacation, they also went on the Memory Prescription Diet, which made it easy for Andrea to stick with her new food choices. Andrea did much better on her exams and was accepted at two of the medical schools to which she applied.

THE 55-YEAR-OLD EXECUTIVE

Elliot R. was proud of his climb up the corporate ladder, but with his new position in a larger company, he felt, for the first time in his life, that he might not be up to the challenge. His talent for remembering names and faces—a skill that he considered key to his success—was slipping. He had always prided himself on knowing every employee's name, and that usually made them feel he was interested and on top of things. But with the move, the new position, and all the other changes, Elliot found himself multitasking and unable to focus. The idea of learning everyone's name was impossible.

The Memory Prescription helped him to get a handle on things. The stress reduction exercises and strategies allowed him to cut back his multitasking so he could pay attention in the moment. He also loved using LOOK, SNAP, CONNECT to help with remembering names and faces.

When Elliot renewed his Prescription, he emphasized the advanced memory training. Not only did he get back his old abilities with names, but he started applying his newly mastered memory techniques to numbers and was having a great time at his family's weekly card games. The stress reduction exercises worked well as an office routine. In the middle of the morning and afternoon each day, he took a 15-minute stress release break that really helped him focus attention. His daily commute didn't leave much time for a physical workout, so he gradually built up his endurance by walking up an additional flight of stairs each week before catching an elevator the rest of the way. His office was on the thirty-eighth floor, which didn't phase him since he was looking forward to a long run at this particular company.

THE 69-YEAR-OLD RETIRED CONTRACTOR

Warren T. had really looked forward to retirement. This was his chance to finally kick back, watch sports for hours on end, and stop worrying about subcontractors. The "no subcontractors" part of his retirement was working out pretty well, but the "limitless spectator sports" thing got old pretty quickly and Warren began feeling bored and fatigued. As a contractor, he had been physically active on his job sites. He knew every trade on each job, and often had to show his guys how he wanted things done. Being glued to the TV set and punching the remote control buttons wasn't cutting it as a workout, but beyond his weekly poker game and occasionally calling some of the guys in the evenings, Warren couldn't motivate himself to get involved in anything new. His boredom and laziness led to a state of forgetfulness and distraction. His wife was fed up and insisted he try something.

The 14-Day Memory Prescription picked up Warren's energy level, and his wife noticed much less forgetfulness. He even remembered her birthday far enough in advance to make reservations for them to get away for the weekend and play golf, which they hadn't done in years. Warren also hadn't realized that the daily challenges of his job had provided a fair degree of mental stimulation, certainly more than he got from the sports channel. He really emphasized the mental aerobics component of his 14-Day Plan and continued to build his mental workout in the months that followed. Warren became a crossword puzzle fanatic and started playing chess again when his son came to visit. He and his wife bought golf clubs and began playing regularly at a local course.

Keeping Your Brain and Body Young for Life

These examples show how people from all walks of life have modified and renewed their program to make it fit in with their particular needs and lifestyle challenges. With this type of approach, every one of us can continue our memory fitness program for years to come, creating lifetime habits and enabling ourselves to achieve quality longevity. You now have the tools that will

help you keep your brain and body young, protect against future memory decline, and delay or possibly even ward off Alzheimer's disease.

The Appendixes that follow include a suggested grocery list, optional
recipes, templates for recording your daily progress, a glossary of terms, and
additional resources offering useful information and services for family members and caregivers. Also, visit my Web site (www.drgarysmall.com) for *Memory Prescription* updates and further information. Good luck and healthy
longevity!

APPENDIX 1:

Suggested Grocery List for the Memory Prescription Diet

Week 1
(Amounts listed are per person)

Fresh Produce
- 1 bunch broccoli
- 1 bunch spinach
- 2 red bell peppers
- 4 large carrots or 1 package baby carrots
- 1 bunch celery
- 1 head Romaine lettuce, 1 butter lettuce
- 1 bunch arugula
- 3 small red potatoes, 1 brown potato
- 1 sweet onion
- 2 zucchinis
- 6 Brussels sprouts
- 2 avocados
- 3 tomatoes
- 2 to 3 cups blueberries
- 1 carton strawberries
- 5 apples
- 1 bunch red grapes
- 3 to 4 bananas
- 3 oranges
- 2 peaches
- 3 pears
- 1 grapefruit
- 2 lemons
- 1 large container raisins
- 1 can/jar each: artichoke hearts, olives, green beans

Dairy
- 1½ dozen eggs
- 6 pint-size containers non-fat yogurt (at least 3 plain)
- 1 pint non-fat milk
- 1 multipack string cheese
- 1 wedge parmesan cheese
- 1 pint low-fat cottage cheese
- 1 package cheddar cheese (shredded or block)
- 1 small container low-fat cream cheese

Meat/Fish

- 3 boneless 6-ounce chicken breasts
- Two 4 to 6 ounce salmon fillets
- One 4 to 6 ounce halibut
- ½ lb ground turkey
- One 4 to 6 ounce sirloin steak
- 1 small package turkey bacon
- 2 to 4 ounces sliced roast beef
- 1 package low-fat turkey dogs
- 2 ounces sliced smoked salmon
- 3 cans tuna (packed in water)

Grains/rice/pasta

- Assorted bread: whole wheat, rye, sourdough; 1 bagel
- 1 package pita bread
- 1 package corn tortillas
- 1 box whole grain crackers
- 1 package oatmeal (regular or instant)
- 1 package brown rice
- 1 box fettuccini

Frozen

- 1 pint frozen yogurt
- 1 pint fruit sorbet
- 1 box frozen fruit bars

Condiments

- 1 jar salsa
- 1 jar natural fruit jam
- 1 bottle olive oil
- 1 bottle balsamic vinegar
- 1 bottle vinaigrette salad dressing

Other

- 6-pack small cans tomato juice
- 2 cans chicken soup with chicken and vegetables
- 2 cans tomato soup
- 8 ounces chopped walnuts
- 4 ounces unsalted peanuts
- 1 small jar natural peanut butter
- 1 package popcorn (for air-popper)
- 1 box tea bags (green is optional)
- 1 to 2 bottles sparkling water if desired
- 1 bottle multivitamins (including 400 mcg folate)
- 1 bottle 500 mgs vitamin C
- 1 bottle 1,000 mgs omega-3 fatty acid supplement
- 1 bottle 400 IUs vitamin E

Week 2

Fresh Produce
- 1 bunch broccoli
- 1 bunch spinach
- 1 red bell pepper
- 3 medium size carrots or 1 package fresh baby carrots
- 1 head Romaine lettuce, 1 butter lettuce (or prewashed bags)
- 1 bunch arugula
- 3 small red potatoes, 1 brown potato
- 1 sweet onion
- 2 zucchinis
- 6 Brussels sprouts
- 2 tomatoes
- 1 to 2 avocados
- 2 to 3 cups blueberries
- 1 carton strawberries
- 5 apples
- 1 bunch red grapes
- 3 to 4 bananas
- 3 oranges
- 2 peaches
- 3 pears
- 1 grapefruit

Dairy
- 1½ dozen eggs
- 6 pint-size containers non-fat yogurt (at least 3 plain)
- 1 pint non-fat milk
- 1 pint low-fat cottage cheese

Meat/Fish
- 3 boneless 6-ounce chicken breasts
- Two 6 to 8 ounce salmon fillets
- One 4 to 6 ounce halibut
- ½ lb ground turkey
- One 4 to 6 ounce sirloin steak
- 2 to 4 ounces sliced roast beef
- 1 to 2 ounces sliced smoked salmon

Grains/rice/pasta
- 1 bagel and assorted breads as needed

Other
- 2 cans chicken soup with chicken and vegetables
- 2 cans tomato soup
- 1 to 2 bottles sparkling water if desired

APPENDIX 2:

Optional Recipes for the Memory Prescription Diet

Baked Corn Tortilla Chips (makes 2 servings)

4 corn tortillas

Preheat oven to 350°.

Cut the tortillas into eighths, and place on a nonstick cookie sheet, or spray cookie sheet with vegetable cooking spray.

Bake until crisp and slightly brown, about 15–20 minutes. Serve with salsa or Hummus Dip.

Banana/Strawberry Yogurt Smoothie

¾ cup strawberry-flavored non-fat yogurt
½ cup non-fat milk

1 small banana
1 teaspoon honey
2–4 frozen strawberries

Combine all ingredients in a blender and blend until smooth.

Pour into a tall glass and enjoy (can be shared in two smaller glasses).

Chicken Cacciatore (makes 4 servings)

1 medium onion finely chopped
1 cup sliced mushrooms
2 teaspoons olive oil
3–4 ounces tomato paste
2 small plum tomatoes, peeled
    and diced

4 skinless, boned chicken breast
    halves
1 teaspoon dried oregano
1 teaspoon dried rosemary
½ cup dry white wine
½ cup dry red wine

Preheat oven to 350°.

In a nonstick skillet, heat the oil and add the garlic, onion, and mushrooms. Stir often until soft, then mix in the tomatoes, oregano, and rosemary.

After a minute, remove from heat and spread mixture in a small baking dish.

Heat the skillet, spray with nonstick vegetable cooking spray, and brown the chicken on both sides.

Place the chicken on top of the tomato mixture in the baking dish, and bake for 10 minutes, covered.

Whisk together the tomato paste and both wines, then pour over chicken. Continue baking for another 20 minutes, covered.

Serve alone or with pasta, and spoon sauce on top of each chicken breast.

Cinnamon Baked Apple (makes 1–2 servings)

1 apple, cored and halved
1 teaspoon apple juice concentrate
    (thawed)

⅛ teaspoon cinnamon

Place apple halves in a glass baking dish and brush with juice concentrate. Sprinkle with cinnamon and bake, covered (microwave: 5 minutes; conventional oven: 45 minutes at 350°).

Remove cover and cool before serving.

Featherweight Cheesecake (makes 10–12 servings)

1 cup plain low-fat yogurt
3 cups low-fat cottage cheese
8 ounces fat-free cream cheese
2 tablespoons orange zest

1 teaspoon lemon zest
Pinch of salt
1/3 cup graham cracker crumbs
1/4 cup chocolate syrup (optional)

Preheat oven to 350°.

Combine all ingredients except chocolate syrup and graham cracker crumbs in a food processor and blend until smooth.

Spray a 10-inch cake pan with nonstick vegetable spray and cover with graham cracker crumbs.

Pour cheese mixture over graham cracker crumbs, and drizzle chocolate syrup on top of cake if desired.

Place cake pan in larger shallow baking pan, and fill larger pan halfway with water. Bake for approximately 1½ hours or until middle of cake is set. Add water to larger pan if level gets low during baking.

Remove cake pan from water and chill.

Hummus Dip (makes about 2 cups)

2½ cups garbanzo beans, drained
1 tablespoon lemon juice
2 cloves garlic, minced
1 tablespoon reduced-fat
    mayonnaise

2 teaspoons tahini
2 teaspoons chopped parsley
½ teaspoon cumin (optional)

Mix all ingredients in a blender or food processor until reaching desired texture.

Chill and serve with baked tortilla chips, pita wedges, or sliced vegetables.

Orange Grove French Toast (makes 4 servings)

2 eggs (or 1 egg plus 2 egg whites)   ¼ teaspoon cinnamon
1 cup orange juice   ¼ cup all-fruit strawberry jam
¼ cup non-fat milk   8 slices whole-grain bread
½ teaspoon sugar

In a bowl, combine ½ cup of the orange juice with the eggs, milk, sugar, and cinnamon.

In a saucepan, whisk together the remaining orange juice and the strawberry jam.

Simmer over low heat, stirring until most of the jam is liquefied.

Coat a nonstick skillet with nonstick cooking spray, and warm over medium heat. Dip one piece of bread at a time into the egg mixture, coating on both sides.

Cook bread in the skillet until both sides are golden brown.

Drizzle with orange-strawberry syrup mixture and enjoy.

Peanut Butter/Ricotta Spread

¼ cup low-fat ricotta cheese   1 tablespoon sugar (or 1 packet
¾ cup low-fat cottage cheese   sugar substitute)
1 tablespoon reduced-fat peanut   1 teaspoon apple juice concentrate
    butter*   (frozen)

Combine all ingredients in food processor and blend until smooth and creamy.

Use as a dip for celery, carrots, or apple slices. Store in refrigerator for up to a week.

*To create natural, reduced-fat peanut butter, buy the non-hydrogenated kind and pour off the oil floating at the top of the jar. To remove even more oil, bunch up a paper towel and stuff it into the top of the jar. Replace the cap, and store upside down in the refrigerator. Replace the paper towel as needed until peanut butter reaches the desired dryness.

Pear Crisp (makes 3–4 servings)

1 cup pears, peeled and sliced
    thinly (or one 8-ounce can
    water-packed pears, drained)
1½ tablespoons flour
1½ tablespoons apple juice
    concentrate (thawed)

⅓ teaspoon cinnamon
Dash of nutmeg
3 tablespoons graham cracker
    crumbs
¾ tablespoon melted margarine

Preheat oven to 375°.

In a small baking dish, toss the pears in ¾ tablespoon flour.

Add apple juice concentrate and coat the pears.

In a bowl, combine spices, crumbs, and remaining flour. Slowly stir in margarine until mixture feels like cookie crumbs. Sprinkle it over the pears.

Bake approximately 30 minutes or until topping is lightly browned.

Turkey and Veggie Chili (makes 4–6 servings)

1 pound ground turkey meat
1 large tomato, diced
1 yellow onion, diced
1 clove garlic, minced
1 red pepper, diced
1 green pepper, diced
1 14.5-ounce can stewed tomatoes
1 cup shredded low-fat cheddar
    cheese (optional)

1 15-ounce can kidney beans—
    drained
1 8-ounce can corn—drained
1 teaspoon chili powder
½ teaspoon cayenne
salt and pepper to taste
2 tablespoons balsamic vinegar
2 teaspoons olive oil
Added water if chili is too thick

Sauté the garlic, onion, and peppers in a nonstick pan using a vegetable cooking spray. Add turkey meat and brown.

Stir in all canned ingredients.

Stir in chili powder, cayenne, salt, and pepper. Blend in balsamic vinegar. Bring mixture to a boil, reduce heat, and simmer for 25 minutes or until chili reaches desired thickness.

Serve in bowls, topped with diced tomatoes and cheddar cheese if desired.

Wild Rice (makes four ½ cup servings)

1½ cups fat-free chicken stock   *½ cup wild rice**
    (canned or fresh)

Before cooking, clean the rice by covering it with cold water and allowing any debris to float to the surface and be removed. Drain well.

In a saucepan, bring the chicken stock to a boil.

Stir in the rice. Cover and reduce heat. Simmer 45–50 minutes or until the rice is tender and the kernels burst.

Remove from stove and fluff rice with fork.

*Wild rice contains the amino acid lysine, not found in most other grains. It is believed to be higher in protein and fiber than white rice. Wild rice has a striking nutty flavor and a chewy texture.

APPENDIX 3:

Sample Worksheets for Daily Progress Reports

The following worksheets may serve as templates for you to track your progress. You may wish to design your own or use other organizational techniques. A variety of computer programs make it easy to create charts and figures such as those included here. You may also want to enter your personal data into a computer program itself each day, to chart your results and then print them out.

Sample Figure

Record the minutes you spend on a particular task each day and then connect the dots to track progress. Write in the name of the activity in the key to the right of the figure. If you are tracking more than one activity on this chart, use a different color pencil or type of line to connect the dots.

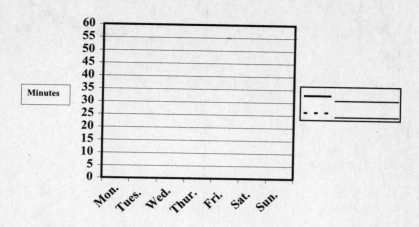

Sample Worksheet

Use the following blank worksheet to create additional worksheets like the ones shown in Chapter 11.

TASK	Mon.	Tues.	Wed.	Thurs.	Fri.	Sat.	Sun.

What to Do If Alzheimer's Disease Strikes

Many of us will be able to use the Memory Prescription to proactively stave off the advance of Alzheimer's and other dementias, as best and long as possible. However, in some cases the genetic risk is high or a person already has several existing risks, such as head injury, high cholesterol, or hypertension, and brain aging may have progressed to the point where it is interfering with daily life. Anyone in this condition should seek professional help.

In *The Memory Bible*, I reviewed the latest information on the diagnosis and treatment of Alzheimer's disease and related dementias. This Appendix is an updated version of that previous information.

Age is the single greatest known risk factor for getting Alzheimer's disease. Approximately 5 percent of people age 65 or older have the disease, but by age 85 that figure soars to between 35 and 47 percent. Advanced brain aging and Alzheimer's disease afflicts over 4 million people in the United States and nearly 25 million people worldwide. Despite such a high prevalence, Alzheimer's disease and other dementias remain under-recognized. Timely recognition is important because treatment is available. Both medication and non-medicinal interventions can slow the progression of the disease and improve functioning in most patients.

Alzheimer's Disease: It's a Family Affair

The devastation of Alzheimer's disease doesn't stop with the patients, it spreads to their families and friends. Watching a loved one decline before your eyes, seeing the personality of someone you cherish gradually disappear, is a traumatic and confusing experience, often leading to anger, sadness, guilt, and depression in the family member and caregiver, as well as the patient. The physical characteristics of a person with Alzheimer's disease remain, but *who* they are eventually vanishes. I have had family members express relief when the patient finally dies, since they have been mourning the loss of that person little by little for years. Research has shown that more than 50 percent of caregivers develop depressions serious enough to require medical intervention. Caregivers miss days at work, have a high risk of becoming physically ill, and often lose sleep, especially when the patient's disease becomes more advanced and is accompanied by agitation and restlessness at night.

A diagnosis of dementia is a staggering consequence for patients and their families, many of whom may have a major economic burden to consider as well as this emotional blow. As baby boomers age over the next few decades, the number of older persons will rise steeply, as too will the cases of Alzheimer's disease. Sadly, by the year 2050, an estimated 14 million Americans will suffer from full-blown Alzheimer's disease. I predict those numbers could be much lower if more people followed at least some of the strategies in *The Memory Prescription*.

Alzheimer's disease is the third most costly disease in the United States, after cardiovascular disease and cancer. Annual costs exceed $100 billion, and most of that is not covered by medical insurance, leaving the families of Alzheimer's patients to bear the greatest economic burden. Earlier intervention in mild to moderate cases can enhance the daily functioning of patients and improve their quality of life. Clearly, keeping our brains young and avoiding symptoms of Alzheimer's disease should be the ultimate goal for all of us.

The Gradual March of Symptoms

Dementia is the general term doctors use to describe loss of memory and other cognitive functions when they impair daily life. With Alzheimer's disease, the course is gradually progressive, memory loss is usually the first symptom to appear, and motor and sensory functions are spared until late stages of the disease. Early on, patients have difficulty learning new information and retaining it for more than a few minutes. As the disease advances, the ability to learn is increasingly compromised, and patients have trouble accessing older, more distant memories. Patients develop problems finding words, using familiar tools and objects, and remaining oriented to time and place.

Eventually, all aspects of their lives become impaired: patients are unable to plan meals, manage finances or medications, use a telephone, and drive without getting lost, and these kinds of difficulties may be the patient's or family's first sign that something is amiss. Social skills usually remain until late in the disease, which contributes, of course, to the delay in recognition of it. As the dementia progresses, judgment becomes impaired, and patients have trouble carrying out even the most basic functions, such as dressing, grooming, and bathing.

Sometimes families have to cope with personality changes, irritability, anxiety, or depression early in the disease, and as the patient worsens, these changes in mood and behavior become more common. Patients lose touch with reality and may become psychotic. They can experience delusions, hallucinations, and aggression, and often wander and get lost. These kinds of behaviors are the most troubling to caregivers, usually distress family members, and lead to nursing home placement.

Alzheimer's disease accounts for approximately 70 percent of dementia cases, while an estimated 15 percent have a condition of motor stiffness and rigidity similar to Parkinson's disease. This combined dementia/Parkinson's syndrome has been termed "dementia associated with Lewy bodies," named for the small round abnormal accumulations found in the patients' brains. Patients with Lewy body dementia often have visual hallucinations and altered alertness. Still another form of dementia strikes primarily the front of the brain and the areas under the temples, so it is known as frontotemporal dementia. These patients often show marked changes in personality and have particular difficulty in executive skills and planning complex tasks, yet their visual and spatial memory tends to be preserved. The cumulative effect of multiple small strokes in the brain causes vascular dementia. Approximately 20 percent of patients with Alzheimer's disease also have vascular disease in the brain.

Many physical illnesses can cause dementia, including infections, cancers that spread to the brain, thyroid disease, or hypoglycemia. Chronic alcohol or drug abuse, as well as a variety of medicines, ranging from antidepressants to antihypertensives, over-the-counter drugs, sleeping pills, and antihistamines, can also cause symptoms of dementia (Chapter 10).

Medical Screening: How the Doctor Checks You Out

When those middle-age pauses are no longer a joke and become a serious matter, that is when Alzheimer's disease can be diagnosed and hopefully recognized early. Too often, physicians and family members accept memory loss, symptoms of depression, and other important diagnostic clues as normal consequences of aging. In the early stages of dementia, I have heard about patients getting into a variety of complications: deeding their house away, being influenced about their will, losing track of substantial sums of money, or marrying a gold digger.

A physician's evaluation of memory loss usually involves an interview, physical examination, and laboratory assessment. In evaluating the patient's mental state, the doctor will screen for depression, memory loss, and other cognitive skills. Laboratory assessments should at least include some blood tests to screen out thyroid disease, vitamin B_{12} deficiency, and other disorders, which could possibly cause memory change.

Doctors often obtain a standardized score of cognitive ability using rating scales like the Mini Mental State Examination, which consists of 30 items that rate memory, orientation, attention, calculation, language, and visual skills. The test takes only about 10 minutes, but is limited because it will not detect subtle memory losses, particularly in college graduates. More detailed memory assessments, known as neuropsychological tests, will provide a better idea about subtle memory deficits.

What's really important to families is how the patient is getting along at home. Dr. Ken Rockwood and his colleagues at Dalhousie University in Nova Scotia have developed a way to measure the patient's response to treatment in terms of how family members and caregivers assess them, focusing on those daily activities they find most important. The doctors created an individualized scale for each patient based upon the family's own descriptions. They ask what drives family members crazy about a patient, then create an outcome measure based on those reports. For example, if Susie T. complained that it drove her crazy when her father asked the same question 20 times a day, Dr. Rockwood might set the six-month treatment goal for Susie's father to asking the same question *only five times* each day.

Brain Scans for Evaluation of Dementia

Some experts recommend computed tomography (CT) or magnetic resonance imaging (MRI), which provide information on the brain's structure. These kinds of scans will detect strokes, brain tumors, or cerebral hemorrhages that occasionally cause symptoms resembling dementia. Unfortunately, in most cases, MRI and CT provide only nonspecific information about brain shrinkage or atrophy or white matter changes, which show up as spots in the deeper brain areas. These changes are often difficult to interpret and rarely provide a diagnosis that will alter treatment.

By contrast, the positron emission tomography (PET) scan is the most effective way to arrive at an early diagnosis. PET enables a physician to make a positive diagnosis of Alzheimer's disease and of other types of dementia, allowing the initiation of anti-dementia drugs, which can improve symptoms and slow the progression of disease while a patient still retains a high level of cognitive function. Early detection also gives patients and their families more time to plan for the future.

At a cost of approximately $1,000 per scan, PET can minimize the need for repetitive diagnostic tests. Depending on the particular clinical setting, such tests can cost upward of $2,000. In the long run, PET scans may save money because earlier diagnosis can eliminate lengthy, costly, and inconclusive evaluations.

PET can identify the Alzheimer's brain pattern months, even years, before obvious symptoms of the disease appear in patients. Dr. Dan Silverman and others in our UCLA research group conducted an international study of nearly 300 patients focusing on the use of PET in the evaluation of dementia. We found that PET scanning is extremely sensitive to early changes and extraordinarily accurate in predicting the future course of dementia. PET demonstrated nearly 95 percent accuracy in predicting the patient's clinical course over three years.

The following images show two-dimensional brain slices with the front of the brain toward the top and the back of the brain toward the bottom. The arrows point to lighter gray areas of decreased brain function.

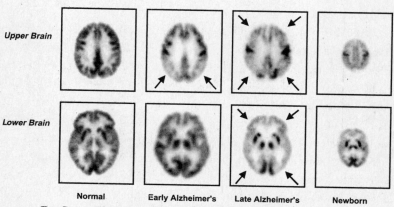

Upper Brain

Lower Brain

Normal   Early Alzheimer's   Late Alzheimer's   Newborn

Pet Scans Showing Function Patterns in a Normal Adult,
an Alzheimer's Patient, and a Newborn

PET reveals a consistent pattern in Alzheimer's disease. Those parietal (arrows in early Alzheimer's) and temporal areas, where Alzheimer's first strikes, show reduced activity in the early stage of the disease. At the late stage, when patients have extreme trouble talking and interacting with others, the frontal areas show decreases. The dark areas midway between the front and back of the advanced Alzheimer's brain control sensation and physical movement and are still at work late in Alzheimer's disease, so these patients are able to experience sensation and control muscle movement. It is remarkable to note that the PET scan of a late stage Alzheimer's patient looks very similar to that of a newborn.

Slowing Decline with Early Treatment

The available cholinergic drugs not only improve memory and other cognitive functions but also benefit overall patient function and help manage some of the behavioral disturbances associated with dementia. Studies show that cholinergic drugs appear to have their greatest therapeutic effect in patients with mild to moderate disease, so early diagnosis is critical in order to help patients maintain the highest level of functioning they have left.

Dr. Murray Raskind, University of Washington, and his collaborators from other U.S. institutions studied what happens when drug treatment is delayed in Alzheimer's patients. They treated half of their volunteers with the cholinesterase inhibitor galantamine (Reminyl), and the other half took a sugar-pill placebo. Six months later, the researchers began giving all the patients the active drug. The group of patients who had been on placebo showed rapid improvement, but they never tested as well as the patients with a six-month jump-start on the medication. In fact, the added benefit for the early starters appeared to continue for the entire year of follow-up, as illustrated below. This apparent benefit of early treatment has been observed in separate studies of the other cholinesterase inhibitor drugs, donepezil (Aricept) and rivastigmine (Exelon).

Six-Month Delay in Cholinergic Treatment

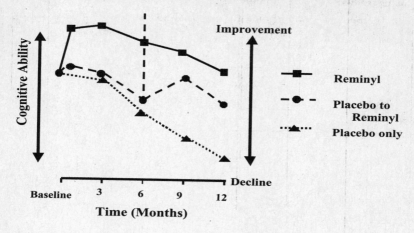

Cholinergic drugs enhance the body's level of acetylcholine, the chemical neurotransmitter that facilitates passage of nerve impulses across synapses. The brains of Alzheimer's patients have a deficiency of acetylcholine, which can result from either impaired production or excess breakdown by enzymes called cholinesterases, and our currently approved treatments inhibit these enzymes, so they are called "cholinesterase inhibitors." Tacrine (Cognex) was the first of these medicines to be approved, but it is now rarely used due to the extent of its side effects. The newer compounds have fewer side effects and include donepezil (Aricept, approved by the FDA in November 1996), rivastigmine (Exelon, approved in April 2000), and galantamine (Reminyl, approved May 2001). These drugs not only improve memory and thinking but they can also reduce agitation and depression. Investigators have been studying their effects on different forms of dementia. Reminyl and Aricept have been shown to be effective in patients with vascular causes of dementia, and Exelon in patients with Lewy body dementia.

Although the majority of patients tolerate these drugs perfectly well, some have reported mild side effects including loss of appetite, indigestion, nausea, slowed heart rate, and insomnia. Most doctors increase the medications gradually in order to minimize side effects, which can occur when the medication is initially begun or the dosage increased. Side effects usually subside with time.

DOSING OF COMMONLY USED CHOLINESTERASE INHIBITORS

Drug	Start Dose	Highest Dose
Donepezil (Aricept)	5 mg, once a day	10 mg, once a day
Rivastigmine (Exelon)	1.5 mg, twice a day	6 mg, twice a day
Galantamine (Reminyl)	4 mg, twice a day	12 mg, twice a day

When beginning cholinergic drug treatment, most patients show improvement, but after months or even a year, they eventually plateau and begin to gradually decline. The big mistake is to assume the drug is no longer working and discontinue treatment once the patient starts this gradual but inevitable decline. But not so fast—the patient *does* have Alzheimer's disease, remember? The drug is meant to treat symptoms and slow further decline. It is *not* a cure. Imagine this patient's decline over a 12-month period without the drug. It would have been much more rapid. So if the patient is tolerating the medicine, stick with it. I advise patients to stay on their medication as long as they are tolerating it since the overwhelming evidence shows that cholinesterase inhibitors can slow the rate of cognitive and functional decline even if patients don't experience obvious initial improvement on the drug.

Alzheimer's patients who take cholinergic drugs need fewer medications for treating depression and behavior problems. They also remain at home and out of nursing homes longer than patients who do not take these medicines.

This past year, a medication that involves a different brain messenger system has become available to patients with Alzheimer's disease. Memantine

(Namenda) works on the brain's NMDA receptors and blocks the brain messenger glutamate in a way that is thought to improve the communication between brain cells. Studies indicate that when 20 milligrams daily are taken, the drug benefits patients with moderate to severe Alzheimer's disease. The drug also may be added to a cholinesterase inhibitor for an additional symptomatic benefit. A recent study found that dementia patients who had been taking Aricept for an average of six months showed additional benefit and slower memory decline when Namenda was added to Aricept, compared with those who remained on Aricept without added Namenda. Like the other available drugs for Alzheimer's disease, it does not cure the disease and eventually patients continue to decline.

Vitamin E for Everybody

If you have been a dutiful follower of the 14-Day Memory Prescription, you have been taking your antioxidant vitamins, including vitamin E, and doing your part to help your body fight those pesky free radicals that wear and tear down your body's DNA. Once Alzheimer's attacks the brain, vitamin E is as important as ever.

Recognizing the potential antioxidant benefits of vitamin E, Dr. Mary Sano, at Columbia University, and her associates found that Alzheimer's patients showed less rapid functional decline if they took 1,000 international units (IUs) of vitamin E twice daily when compared to patients on placebo. Functional decline was defined as amount of time—days, weeks, months— before the patient needed nursing home care, as well as other practical indicators of daily function.

The scientists chose a very high dose of vitamin E to ensure that enough was present to have an effect. Because such high doses could occasionally suppress immune function and the patient's ability to ward off some infections, not all physicians recommend such high doses, preferring 800 to 1,000 IUs per day for patients suffering from Alzheimer's disease. As I mentioned in Chapter 7, I recommend 400 IUs once or twice daily for everyone as a preventative measure.

Treating Behavior Disturbances

Behavior changes in patients with advanced Alzheimer's disease can drive family members and caregivers to depression and their own health problems. If you are caring for someone who constantly yells at you or strikes out or watches you suspiciously all day, it is hard not to react with anger, guilt, or sadness. Unfortunately, caregivers often take the patient's behaviors personally and interpret it as willful rather than resulting from misfiring neurons. These kinds of behavioral changes are what usually lead to the placement of Alzheimer's patients in nursing homes. Caregivers just can't take it anymore.

Sometimes medications will improve symptoms, and non-medicinal approaches can make a big difference. When counseling caregivers on dealing with some of these problems, I often remind them of how we deal with young children. Similar strategies are useful in both situations: simplify communications, distract them when they get frustrated, and maintain a calm but firm attitude.

Antipsychotic drugs are often used to treat psychotic symptoms and agitation in patients with dementia. Newly developed antipsychotics are preferred, including risperidone (Risperdal), quetiapine (Seroquel), olanzapine (Zyprexa), and ziprasidone (Geodon). These newer drugs cause fewer side effects than older antipsychotics like haloperidol (Haldol) or chlorpromazine (Thorazine). For symptoms of anxiety and agitation, the antianxiety drugs are often used. Most physicians prefer the newer drugs, including lorazepam (Ativan), alprazolam (Xanax), and oxazepam (Serax), because older drugs like diazepam (Valium) and chlordiazepoxide (Librium) tend to accumulate in the blood and cause side effects like daytime sedation, unsteady gait, and confusion. The newer drugs will get in and out of the body more quickly and tend to cause fewer side effects.

Some medicines used to treat epilepsy, the anticonvulsants—particularly carbamazepine (Tegretol) and divalproex sodium (Depakote)—represent another group of drugs that shows promise as effective treatments for behavioral problems in demented patients. Dr. Pierre Tariot at the University of Rochester has led the field in using these drugs in this patient population and finds that agitated and aggressive patients who have a manic appearance of rapid thinking and irritability are especially responsive to anticonvulsant medications. For demented patients who develop depression, antidepressants are often prescribed (Chapter 10).

Meeting the Challenges When Things Get Tough

If you are a caregiver, you may want to consider joining a support group to help answer your questions, make you feel less alone, and diminish your level of stress. Feelings of anger, frustration, and guilt are a normal part of caring for a relative or friend or patient with dementia. Community resources can offer some respite care, giving relatives and friends a chance to care for themselves, go to the gym, join a support group, see friends, and other personal activities to recharge their batteries.

Dr. Mary Mittelman and her colleagues at New York University have studied how education and emotional support for caregivers of Alzheimer's patients may delay the patient's placement into nursing homes. They found that the caregivers' education and support had a definite impact on their patients, delaying nursing home placement up to a year.

Establishing a daily routine for patients will improve their behavior and mood. The predictability gives them a sense of security. Clocks and calendars help keep patients oriented. Consider setting up an exercise program that allows patients to move about freely for as long as possible. Newspapers, radios, and televisions are great ways for patients to try to stay up on current events and keep links to the outside world. Try to help them maintain social and intellectual activities and continue to attend family events whenever possible.

If behavior becomes troublesome, try to understand what provokes it. Some patients' symptoms get worse toward the evening, when rooms tend to darken. Other times a particular family member, friend, caregiver, or situation brings on aggressive outbursts. When possible, modify a situation to avoid provocation. Unfortunately, many patients become agitated out of mere frustration, or conversations become too complex, or perhaps they forget the content of the discussion. Try to use simple sentence structure and reassure the patient by gently reminding them of the content of the discussion. If the caregiver can stay calm, the patient often picks up on their composure, which can help them to calm down as well.

For patients who tend to wander, using night-lights and perhaps even raising doorknobs up high may help to keep them safe. Regular supervised walks will promote exercise and may cut down on wandering. However, if a large yard is available so the patient has the space to walk about safely, medications or other forms of restraint can be reduced or avoided. Also contact the Alzheimer's Association (800-272-3900) for information and to register with the SAFE RETURN program, which provides patient name tags and medical-alert bracelets that can help to locate lost patients.

The cognitive impairments of Alzheimer's disease diminish driving skills, and even mildly demented patients often should not be driving, due to their difficulties with visual and spatial skills as well as in planning ahead. Some states, such as California, require the physician to report patients with Alzheimer's disease to better monitor their driving skills. A diagnosis of dementia should clearly raise concern about a person's driving abilities, and patients with advanced dementia should not be driving at all.

The overall goal of caregiving is to maintain the kindest, least restrictive environment as possible, for as long as possible. For many families, this means keeping patients at home and out of long-term care facilities unless it becomes absolutely necessary.

The Memory Prescription for Alzheimer's Victims

The Memory Prescription was designed for people to boost their memory performance and brain health and prevent future cognitive decline leading to Alzheimer's disease and related dementias. However, many of the strategies can be applied, sometimes with modifications, to improve the quality of life of Alzheimer's victims. For advanced dementia, the impact will be minimal. However, most families want to do whatever they can to improve the health and welfare of their loved ones, and these strategies will likely benefit patients with milder forms of dementia. Here are some considerations if you wish to focus on the Big 4 to help a friend or relative with dementia.

Stress Reduction
Alzheimer's patients often experience stress, but at times it can be a challenge to determine its source. One approach is to consider sources of stress from earlier days when the patient's mental faculties were intact. If the patient hated loud music and cigarette smoke then, chances are that they still feel that way, and fresh air and Mozart might calm them down.

Regular physical activity can be a helpful relaxation strategy for patients, especially those who develop motor restlessness as a side effect to medicines used to reduce agitation. Yoga, tai chi, or related exercises that release both physical and mental stress may be effective relaxation techniques for patients with milder cognitive losses, but may be too challenging for patients with advanced dementia.

Even patients with moderate dementia will respond to guided relaxation exercises to help them focus on deep breathing and calm settings. When the instructions are simple and clear, they can follow along and enjoy the quieting effects. Most patients, however, would be unable to initiate such exercises on their own. Professional treatments like massage therapy may also help to reduce anxiety and stress, particularly if the patient enjoyed such treatments before the onset of dementia.

Memory Prescription Diet
The Memory Prescription Diet is based on the latest scientific findings indicating dietary strategies that promote brain and body fitness. Patients with dementia also would benefit from its goals: moderate caloric intake, ample portions of omega-3 fatty acids, antioxidant-rich foods, and low glycemic index carbohydrates. Encouraging frequent meals will also help to stabilize blood sugar levels, which could minimize agitation in some patients. Excessive liquids may need to be avoided in dementia patients who suffer from urinary incontinence.

Physical Activity

Patients with dementia do well with routine physical activity, which will help them to maintain cardiac and brain health through improved circulation. For patients who have prior experience with aerobic conditioning, returning to their familiar exercise routine is often an effective approach, rather than trying out new forms of aerobic workout. Patients may benefit from such fitness toys as treadmills or weight machines, but they often require supervision and assistance from others. Patients with impaired memory and other cognitive functions do best when activities are planned and part of a daily routine. A regular evening walk can be a nice way for both the caregiver and the patient to get out together and get some exercise.

Mental Activity

Several neuroscientists have begun developing intensive mental stimulation interventions designed to arouse brain cell function and improve cognitive abilities in patients with dementia. The rationale for this approach is based on the same scientific literature suggesting that such stimulation will protect neurons and keep them healthy longer. Some even speculate that intensive mental aerobics for patients with dementia would trigger neural repair to some extent.

Families and clinicians have reported that when the mental activity is at the right level of difficulty, patients with dementia appear to benefit. When working with families, I suggest that they try leisure activities that the patient enjoyed before the impairment. For example, the son of a 78-year-old man with vascular dementia found that his father's mental acuity and personality lit up when the two of them played billiards together, a game that they both enjoyed over many years. Another 73-year-old woman enjoyed golf before she developed Alzheimer's disease. Although she was no longer able to negotiate the full 18 holes at the club, her caregiver brought her out to a miniature golf course where she spent hours enjoying the putting. Some clinicians have their patients read aloud from Hardy Boys or Nancy Drew books or any material that is at the level of a younger reader. Both the patients and the caregivers enjoy the readings.

Memory training techniques are generally not recommended for patients with dementia because they are usually too challenging and patients become frustrated. Instead, practical strategies for helping patients cope with their cognitive losses (e.g., daily routines, orienting measures, calendars, labels, etc.) can help maximize the patient's limited cognitive abilities.

What to Do If Alzheimer's Disease Strikes

- Seek professional help in attaining an accurate diagnosis so appropriate treatment can begin sooner rather than later.
- Ask the doctor about medication treatments, including cholinergic drugs and vitamin E. Discuss other practical and legal issues with the doctor.
- Join a support group for family members and caregivers through the Alzheimer's Association or local community groups where available.
- Expect that the patient's behavior will change over time and may become difficult. Remember that these changes are not willful but are a result of a physical brain disease.
- Maintain the patient's social and family activities as much as and as long as possible.
- Individualize sensory input to the patient's needs.
- Try to understand the cause of a patient's troublesome behavior and attempt to avoid it.
- Keep daily activities routine and surroundings familiar.
- Arrange a regular exercise schedule to promote fitness and minimize wandering. If necessary and possible, provide an environment where the patient can wander safely.
- Display clocks and calendars to help orient the patient.

- For the safety of the patient as well as everyone on the road, patients with moderate to severe dementia should not drive under any circumstances.
- Many of the stress reduction, healthy diet, physical conditioning, and mental activity strategies of the Memory Prescription will benefit patients with dementia.

APPENDIX 5:

Research Update and
What's on the Horizon

The near future will surely bring many new approaches to keeping our brains and bodies young. It may be possible one day to drive to the local shopping mall and take a seat in the waiting room of a quality longevity center. Soon an anti-aging technician could hook us up to a portable scanner that in about three minutes will determine the plaque and tangle buildup in our key brain memory centers, indicating our current extent of brain aging. Then, after providing a mere strand of our hair for full-body genetic-risk analysis, the technician feeds this information into a computer, factors in our age, height, weight, and other key bits of data, and almost instantly prints out a two-page program instructing us on what anti-aging medicines, hormones, supplements, and preventive measures we ought to take for us to achieve our healthy longevity target. Most of us will probably anticipate living to anywhere from 110 to 130 years, depending on individual genetic advantages or disadvantages.

Many experts are convinced that we can reach that goal, and some individuals already do so without the benefit of future drugs and vaccines that will likely improve everyone's chances. Dr. Karen Ritchie reported on a woman from the South of France, who died at the age of 122. The woman's autopsy revealed the brain of a healthy 80-year-old. Dr. Ritchie noted that her patient probably had a genetic advantage—her relatives survived several lethal influenza epidemics. But she also lived the healthy brain and body lifestyle: plenty of physical and mental activity and a Mediterranean diet known to promote brain and body health.

I am convinced that in the next five to ten years, we will witness major breakthroughs in achieving quality longevity. Innovative scientists throughout the world are applying new technologies that will make huge differences in the average life span and, more important, in the quality of life we enjoy. The prospect of becoming "senile and wasting away in a nursing home" will hopefully develop into a scenario of past generations.

A New Peek into Brain Windows

The outward, physical signs of aging are obvious, as my nine-year-old son recently noted when he asked if I had started "dyeing my hair white." However, brain aging is not so obvious. In fact, it wasn't until recent years that medical technology finally advanced scanning methods to the extent that we could see into the brain and recognize the subtle evidence of brain aging and the early indications of Alzheimer's disease.

Doctors are becoming more familiar with positron emission tomography, which allows us to visualize how well brain cells function. In fact, in the United States, Medicare pays for PET scans to assist with diagnosis and treatment of many cancers and heart conditions. As of this writing, such benefits are not yet available to assist in the diagnosis of dementia. However, the available scientific evidence shows us that PET scanning does help with early diagnosis of Alzheimer's disease, often years before most doctors would be able to confirm the diagnosis with conventional methods. In a brain PET scan of someone with mild cognitive losses, a doctor may see reduced activity in the parietal and temporal brain areas—the areas where Alzheimer's first strikes (Appendix 4). These scans guide physicians to begin treating patients with anti-Alzheimer's medications sooner than they might have without the scan, thus providing the patient the added value of early treatment.

Our research group at UCLA also has discovered another way to use the

PET scanner. Rather than simply visualizing how well the brain cells are communicating, our newly developed technology lets us view directly the Alzheimer's amyloid plaques and tangles as they accrue in the brains of living people, thus avoiding the unnecessary delay, trauma, and, of course, death that is required by the conventional method of viewing these brain lesions only at autopsy. This recent discovery not only provides investigators a way to monitor new drugs for treating and preventing Alzheimer's disease, but it could help us detect the disease earlier and get a jump on thwarting it altogether.

My research partner, Dr. Jorge Barrio, a UCLA professor and chemist, has synthesized several novel molecules that work as chemical markers of the disease in the brain. Barrio adds a radioactive label to the markers so we can measure a signal reflecting the extent of this plaque buildup in different brain regions, with the help of the PET scanner. The initial results are striking. We see a heavy signal in the very areas of the brain where autopsy studies show that the plaques and tangles accumulate. And the technique may pick up the subtle presence of amyloid plaques in people even before they develop obvious symptoms of dementia. The signal appears greater in healthy individuals who have a genetic risk for Alzheimer's disease compared with those who have no known genetic risk. Volunteers with just mild memory complaints also have a higher PET scan signal if they have lower scores on memory tests.

Our group is currently working with other researchers to use this new form of PET scanning to study medications being developed to wipe out plaques and tangles. International enthusiasm for this technology is considerable since it promises to streamline drug discovery, particularly for treatments designed to slow and possibly eliminate age-related cognitive decline and Alzheimer's disease.

Other exciting brain imaging work involves magnetic resonance imaging scanners that are used extensively today for diagnosing strokes, brain tumors, or blood clots. Our research team and others have altered the MRI method so the scans can measure regional brain activity from moment to moment while volunteers perform memory tasks (Chapter 1). This brain stress test shows us how our brains work harder to compensate for subtle deficits. Other studies use the MRI scan to measure concentrations of chemical markers in the brain that reflect brain cell function as well as the integrity of the connections between the neurons. In the future, we will likely use a combination of brain imaging techniques to best predict when our brains will begin to age and how early we ought to intervene.

Genetic Keys to Better Brain Health

The science of genetics has ballooned during the past two decades. Most of us know that genes are the blueprints of life, and our DNA defines our individuality.

When we think of genetic traits being passed from one generation to the next, we usually think of physical features such as hair and eye color, facial features, height and build, and so on. It is only in recent years that medical conditions such as heart disease, high cholesterol, and cancer have been discovered to pass within families genetically.

Traditionally, the common, late-onset form of Alzheimer's disease, which affects people after age 65, was not thought to have a genetic influence, but to be a normal result of aging. We now believe the cause involves a combination of environmental, lifestyle, and genetic influences.

Many genes have been discovered to be involved with age-related memory loss and Alzheimer's disease. A defect in some genes causes early-onset familial Alzheimer's, a rare and devastating form of the disease that hits people early in life, before age 65, and normally strikes half the relatives in those families.

For the common late-onset Alzheimer's, however, one major genetic risk has been discovered: apolipoprotein E or APOE. This APOE gene makes a protein that transports cholesterol and fats through the body and is known to influence the risk for heart disease and related conditions. APOE comes in three different forms: APOE-2, APOE-3, and APOE-4. All of us inherit one APOE form from each parent for a combination of two forms, known as a genotype. APOE-4 is much more frequent in Alzheimer's patients than in normal people. Approximately 65 percent of the population has the APOE ⅔ genotype, 25 percent has the ¾ genotype—a high risk for developing late-onset Alzheimer's disease—and 2 percent has the ¼ genotype—an even higher risk for Alzheimer's disease.

Although the APOE-4 gene increases a person's risk for Alzheimer's and makes it more likely that they'll get the disease at a younger age, an APOE blood test result alone is not enough to accurately predict whether an individual will get the disease. And we know that APOE accounts for only about half of the total genetic risk for most people, so other genes are involved.

Scientists are searching for additional genes that increase or decrease an individual's risk for developing rapid brain aging or dementia. Such genetic variants will probably help us identify the best candidate for a memory enhancing drug or treatment to prevent dementia. Particular genetic variants may lead to differences in an individual's drug response, so doctors may eventually know a patient's drug response profile before beginning medication treatment. The point is to avoid unnecessarily treating patients whose genetics indicate they may receive little benefit from a given drug yet have a high risk for side effects.

Vaccine Update: Don't Give Up Hope

Several years ago, an Irish drug company named Elan Pharmaceuticals was in the news because they had developed a vaccine that appeared to successfully treat mice with human Alzheimer's disease. The vaccine was developed to clear out the presumably toxic amyloid plaques that build up in the Alzheimer's brain in key memory regions.

In an approach that differed from other pharmaceutical companies, the Elan scientists manufactured a synthetic form of the protein building block that eventually accumulates to form the insoluble amyloid plaque. In these experiments, the protein vaccine created a heightened immune response that sloughs off the plaque deposits leading to Alzheimer's disease. The immune system, or the body's mechanism for fighting off disease, recognizes antigens or foreign bodies and responds with antibodies designed to search and destroy the foreigner.

Dr. Dale Schenk and his associates at Elan found that monthly injections of this protein raised the level of antibodies that the brain produced and actually prevented Alzheimer's disease–type brain degeneration in young Alzheimer's transgenic mice—mice that were genetically programmed to produce the amyloid-beta that creates the sticky plaques of the disease. Remarkably, the injections also eliminated plaques in older mice by as much as 80 percent. The vaccine improved their cognitive ability to master a maze.

Despite the enthusiasm for these experiments, skeptics warned that we don't yet know if the memory loss associated with Alzheimer's disease will significantly improve following depletion of the amyloid plaques, and it is possible that immunization with amyloid-beta may simply clear the plaques from the brain and have only minimal effects on memory loss. At the end of the treatment, the good news may be that you have no brain plaques; the bad news could be that you might not recall the doctor telling you the good news.

The only surefire way to know if the vaccine effectively treats the disease is to test it in humans in a large-scale, double-blind placebo test. The excitement for the human studies was so high that not only were volunteers put on long waiting lists to get into the clinical trials, but many of the clinics testing the vaccine were kept anonymous to cope with the continuous onslaught of eager volunteers. In early 2002, nearly 400 patients were enrolled in these vaccine trials when, unfortunately, the company had to pull the plug on the study because the vaccine caused a life-threatening brain inflammation leading to swelling and confusion.

Currently, scientists are scrambling to create novel and safe versions of an Alzheimer's vaccine. If current efforts succeed, we might see an Alzheimer's vaccine on the market in the next five years. The pursuit is fueled by preliminary findings that in patients who made the key antibodies and did not suffer from brain inflammation, memory decline either stabilized or improved during the one-year study. In two of the patients, memory scores returned to normal levels, suggesting that a safe vaccine strategy could even reverse existing brain damage. One promising strategy for revamping the vaccine involves injecting patients with laboratory manufactured antibody instead of the protein vaccine to stimulate a natural antibody response. These synthetic antibodies may work just as well and are not likely to cause the brain inflammation.

Better Living Through Smart Drugs

Had a long, tough day at the office and feeling too fuzzy-headed to help Junior with his algebra homework? Cramming for final exams and worried this test will keep you from getting into Harvard Business School? Up too late last night and afraid of blowing this morning's pitch meeting? Some day you may be able to meet these mental challenges by simply walking to your medicine cabinet and choosing between a variety of "smart drug" tablets to boost your brain power for the next few hours, days, or the rest of your life (depending on your dosage and body weight, of course).

Science is already heading in this direction. Off-label use of existing anti-Alzheimer's drugs, as well as development of new medications, are being looked at to try and boost brain power as well as slow down the brain's march towards Alzheimer's disease.

By the time a patient develops Alzheimer's disease symptoms, the damage to their brain has already occurred. This and other evidence has convinced me that our best chance of "curing" Alzheimer's disease is to target mild forgetfulness. At UCLA, we are conducting double-blind studies using an individual's genetic risk profile to help us track over time how well a particular medication treatment is slowing down brain aging and delaying the onset of Alzheimer's disease. All research subjects are tested for any APOE-4 Alzheimer's genetic risk. They also receive a PET scan before starting treatment as well as a follow-up scan two years later. We predict that the volunteers who take placebo pills will show more rapid decline in brain function (i.e., accelerated brain aging) than those taking an active drug. We expect the actual drug to be more effective in volunteers with the APOE-4 genetic risk than those without the genetic risk. Our aim is to delay brain aging by one or more decades, thus allowing people to live longer, and better, without memory decline.

The type of drug or vaccine we wish to test will determine the type of brain imaging technology we use to track our progress. If our drug is designed to clear out plaques, then we'll use our plaque PET scanner. If we think we will have our greatest drug effect on brain efficiency, then the functional MRI brain stress test will give us the best results. These techniques allow us to study fewer people in less time than we would if we only employed the standard pencil and paper memory tests.

This line of research also raises the possibility of improving our brain power even if we have nothing wrong with it. Some contend that this "Viagra for the brain" approach is "cheating" or "cheap." Yet use of drugs such as cognitive enhancers has been a part of our lifestyle ever since our ancestors first enjoyed a cup of coffee. As we learned in Chapter 10, many new drugs, hormones, and supplements are in development and being considered for testing for use as possible "smart drugs." Some of the new drugs in the pipeline aim to boost the brain's ability to form memories despite the existence of plaques and tangles. A group of drugs called ampakines increase the activity of brain chemicals important to memory formation. Ampakines are being tested in patients with Alzheimer's disease as well as people with only mild cognitive impairment.

Other studies have found that cholinesterase inhibitor drugs used to treat Alzheimer's disease may in fact improve cognitive performance in healthy individuals. Dr. Jerry Yesavage of Stanford University and Dr. Peter Whitehouse of Case Western Reserve University and their colleagues trained a group of pilots in a Cessna 172 simulator. During the training, one group of pilots took the drug donepezil (Aricept) and the other took a placebo. A month after the initial training, they gave the pilots a challenging session testing their training recall, with lots of complicated air-traffic maneuvers and tasks requiring emergency reactions. The pilots on Aricept performed significantly better than the pilots taking placebos.

Additional drugs stimulate the production and release of growth factors in the brain's memory centers. Such growth factors coax nerve cells to create new connections with each other. Some pharmaceutical companies are developing experimental drugs that enhance the activity and possible growth of undamaged neurons in the brain's memory centers. Even if a successful approach is developed to eliminate plaque buildup, patients will still need to have treatment of memory problems. Thus, one medicine or course of treatment may affect disease progression while another improves function.

As newer technologies emerge in the next decade, I predict ever more profound breakthroughs to halt the relentless advance of brain aging. It is likely that we will be using these approaches not just to slow down the process but to improve our cognitive functioning to the limit. In the meantime, I am sticking with my non-pharmacological Memory Prescription to keep *my* brain young. And you should too.

APPENDIX 6:

Glossary

Acetylcholine. A neurotransmitter involved in memory, learning, and concentration. The cholinergic neurons that produce brain acetylcholine decline in normal aging and in Alzheimer's disease.

Acetyl-l-carnitine. Acetyl-l-carnitine promotes the neurotransmitter acetylcholine and may protect brain neurons. Some human studies show a benefit over placebo for memory performance.

Active observation. The process of focusing attention so that new information is stored into memory.

Aerobic exercise. Exercise that gets the heart pumping faster and the lungs breathing deeper so more oxygen is delivered to the body's cells. Examples of aerobic exercise include calisthenics, rapid walking, jogging, and swimming. Research suggests that aerobic conditioning benefits brain function in the frontal lobe.

Age-associated memory impairment. The term for the common memory changes that accompany normal aging, defined as a memory change demonstrated by at least one standard memory test, along with a subjective awareness of memory changes.

Age-related cognitive decline. A condition of noticeable decline in mental ability without the presence of disease.

Alzheimer's disease. The most common form of dementia. Its onset is gradual and course progressive. The physician can make a "probable" diagnosis, but a "definite" diagnosis is made only through autopsy or biopsy.

Ampakines. Drugs that increase the activity of brain chemicals important to memory formation. Ampakines are being tested in patients with Alzheimer's disease and mild cognitive impairment.

Amyloid plaques. Collections of abnormal insoluble protein, present in high concentrations in the areas involved in memory in the Alzheimer's brain.

Amyloid-beta. A small molecule consisting of about 40 amino acids strung together like a beaded necklace. Amyloid-beta is the building block of the insoluble protein that forms the core of Alzheimer's plaques, thought to be toxic to the brain.

Anti-amyloid vaccine. A synthetic form of amyloid-beta used to vaccinate mice that have been genetically engineered to form the Alzheimer's plaques.

Antioxidants. Drugs, vitamins, or foods that interfere with oxidative stress.

Apolipoprotein E (APOE). A gene on chromosome 19 that comes in three different forms (2, 3, and 4). One copy of the APOE-4 gene increases the risk for Alzheimer's disease and lowers the average age when people first develop symptoms. Two copies have the same effect, but more so.

Brain stress test. An experimental method to tease out subtle brain abnormalities. Volunteers perform memory tasks while a functional MRI scanner measures brain activity response to memory performance.

Cholinesterase inhibitors. Drugs approved by the FDA for the treatment of Alzheimer's disease. These drugs inhibit the cholinesterase enzymes, which break down acetylcholine, resulting in an increase in acetylcholine and improved cognition in patients. Current investigations are focusing on their potential for treating milder forms of memory loss and delaying the onset of Alzheimer's disease.

Clioquinoline. This antibiotic was once used to treat traveler's diarrhea and is now under investigation as a possible anti-amyloid treatment for Alzheimer's disease. Tests in transgenic Alzheimer's mice indicate clioquinoline attaches to the metals in the brain plaques and clears them out, leading to more than a 50-percent reduction in plaques, as well as improved general behavior. Scientists have begun comparing the drug with placebo in patients with Alzheimer's disease.

Coenzyme Q_{10}. An antioxidant supplement that has been used to treat age-related memory loss or to slow the progression of Alzheimer's disease, although systematic research is limited. The supplement can interact with medicines used to treat heart failure, diabetes, and kidney or liver problems.

Cognition (cognitive function). Mental function involving memory, language abilities, visual and spatial skills, intelligence, and reasoning.

Computerized tomography (CT) scan. A computer-enhanced X-ray that provides pictures of brain structure that can assist in the diagnosis of brain tumors, strokes, and blood clots.

Coronary heart disease. Heart disease caused by a buildup of plaque in the coronary blood vessels, which provide blood and nutrients to the heart muscles.

Cortisol. A stress hormone secreted by the adrenal glands. Chronically high levels of cortisol can impair memory performance.

Cox II inhibitors. A group of anti-inflammatory drugs that inhibit only one of the enzymes (cyclooxygenase II) involved in inflammation. These drugs have fewer side effects than older cyclooxygenase inhibitors, which inhibit both cox I and cox II enzymes and are more likely to cause gastric bleeding. These drugs are currently being studied as treatments to prevent Alzheimer's disease.

Creatine. A dietary supplement that has been used to enhance sports performance and reduce fatigue. Initial results from new research indicates potential cognitive benefits as well.

Curcumin. The active ingredient in turmeric, curcumin has anti-inflammatory and antioxidant actions. It has been used in patients with arthritis and is currently being tested as a treatment for cognitive decline.

Dehydropeindrosterone (DHEA). The body converts DHEA into estrogen and testosterone. DHEA supplements may strengthen the immune system and heighten sex drive and activity level. Side effects include an increased risk for prostate cancer, facial hair growth, scalp balding, and acne. Studies of its potential memory benefits are inconclusive.

Dementia. Impairment in memory and at least one other cognitive function (e.g., language, visual-spatial skill) to the extent that it interferes with daily life.

Dendrites. Short, branching extensions of neurons that receive impulses from other neurons when neurotransmitters stimulate them.

Dimethylaminoethanol (DMAE). A dietary supplement that boosts the brain's cholinergic messenger system. Until the early 1980s, it was used to treat behavior and learning problems in children with attention deficits and has since become available as a dietary supplement.

DL-Phenylalanine. A combination of essential amino acids used to promote mental functioning, mood, and muscle relaxation.

Donepezil (Aricept). A cholinesterase inhibitor drug used to treat Alzheimer's disease. Donepezil should be increased from 5 to 10 mg daily after six weeks. Dose increases should be slower if patients have difficulties tolerating side effects.

Endorphins. Hormones responsible for the mild euphoria we feel after aerobic exercise, often described as the body's own internal circulating antidepressant.

Enzyme. A protein that controls chemical reactions in the body.

Epidemiological studies. Studies of large numbers of participants that count up rates of disease and factors that might influence disease risk.

Estrogen. Current studies will determine if estrogen replacement therapy after menopause lowers the risk for Alzheimer's disease. Taking estrogen along with progestin increases the risk for dementia. Studies of estrogen as a treatment for Alzheimer's disease have been disappointing, and it is not recommended for treating memory loss.

Executive control. Cognitive abilities such as planning, scheduling, coordination, and actively inhibiting information, generally mediated in the frontal and prefrontal brain regions.

Free radicals. Ubiquitous molecules, also known as oxidants, present in the air we breathe, the food we eat, and the water we drink. Free radicals cause oxidative stress and wear down the genetic material, or DNA, of our cells. This process accelerates aging and contributes to chronic diseases such as cancer and Alzheimer's.

Frontal lobe. The front part of the brain that mediates executive control.

Galantamine (Reminyl). A cholinesterase inhibitor drug used to treat Alzheimer's disease. Galantamine treatment should begin at 4 mg twice daily and increase every month for a maximum dose of 12 mg twice daily. Dose increases should be slower if patients have difficulties tolerating side effects.

Genes. The blueprint for life contained in all the body's cells, inherited from parents, and consisting of deoxyribonucleic acid (DNA). The molecular configuration of the double-helical strands of DNA is an alphabet key, a genotype, that programs our phenotype—who we are mentally and physically. A minute molecular change can have a dramatic effect on a person's risk for a particular disease.

Ginkgo biloba. A Chinese herb used to treat memory loss. Previous studies suggesting a benefit have not yet been confirmed.

Glucose. A simple sugar that is the main source of energy in the body's cells and results from the break down of foods we eat.

Glycemic index. A measure of how rapidly a food causes blood sugar levels to rise. This index ranks foods from 0 to 100, indicating whether the food raises blood sugar levels gradually (low scores) or rapidly (high scores).

Gram (gm). A measurement used for drugs equivalent to 1/28 of an ounce.

Growth hormone stimulants. These natural products trigger the release of chemical messengers to increase growth hormone secretion. The stress reducing effects of growth hormone suggest a possible role for these compounds, though minimal evidence supports any memory benefits.

Hippocampus. A seahorse-shaped brain structure involved in memory and learning, located in the temporal lobe of the brain (near the temples).

Huperzine A. A dietary supplement that inhibits cholinesterase enzyme. Although not all studies have been positive, huperzine appears to benefit patients with dementia and people with mild states of memory loss.

Hormones. Chemical messengers produced by glands and organs in the body and absorbed into the bloodstream.

Hydergine. Derived from a rye fungus, hydergine acts on several neurotransmitters that influence memory. It has been used extensively as a cognitive enhancer throughout the world. Studies of patients with dementia or with age-associated cognitive symptoms have yielded mixed results.

Hypercholesterolemia. Elevated blood levels of cholesterol. A risk factor for diseases affecting blood vessels in the heart, brain, and other body organs.

Hypertension (high blood pressure). A chronic disease that increases risk for circulatory problems, heart disease, and vascular dementia.

Immediate memory. Fleeting memories for sights, sounds, and other stimuli that last for milliseconds before moving into short-term memory.

Immune response. The body's mechanism for developing a memory for foreign or threatening materials or organisms. Specialized immune cells are primed initially so they will quickly produce antibodies to ward off infection. The immune system recognizes and destroys proteins such as insoluble amyloid beta that are not normally present.

Inflammation. The body's natural response to infection or stress, consisting of a mobilization of specialized cells to eliminate the offending foreign body.

Insulin. A hormone produced by the pancreas that gets sugar into cells.

Insulin resistance. The inability of cells to respond to insulin, resulting in high blood sugar levels.

Ischemia. Lack of oxygen to body tissue. In the brain, it can have several effects: if brief, it leads to transient ischemic attacks (TIAs) when the patient has a temporary loss of memory or motor function. When prolonged, it leads to death of brain cells and permanent deficits, known as strokes or cerebral vascular accidents (CVAs).

Lecithin. A major component of all living cells, lecithin is broken down in the body to active cholinergic compounds that have minimal but inconsistent memory benefits. The average diet contains about a gram of lecithin, and tenfold greater amounts are used as supplements given in daily divided doses.

Lesion. Any damage to body tissues or cells.

Linking. A memory technique that associates or connects two or more bits of information.

Long-term memory. Relatively permanent memory that has been organized and rehearsed.

LOOK, SNAP, CONNECT. A basic three-step memory technique that includes (1) actively observing what you want to learn (*LOOK*), (2) creating mental snapshots of memories (*SNAP*), and (3) linking mental snapshots together (*CONNECT*).

Lycopene. A potent antioxidant present in high concentrations in tomatoes.

Magnetic resonance imaging (MRI) scan. A brain scanning technique providing more detailed information on brain structure than CT scanning. MRI can be useful in diagnosing brain tumors, strokes, and blood clots. When modified, it can produce information on brain function, a technique known as functional MRI.

Major depression. A serious form of depression that can interfere with memory ability.

Melatonin. The principal hormone secreted by the pineal gland, melatonin is a brain messenger with a structure similar to serotonin. The hormone regulates mood, sleep, sexual behavior, reproductive alterations, immunologic function, and the sleep-wake cycle. Its antioxidant activity has led investigators to consider it as a treatment against Alzheimer's disease.

Memantine (Namenda). A drug that acts on the N-methyl-D-aspartate (NMDA) brain receptor involved in memory function. The number of these receptors decreases in Alzheimer's disease, and recent studies indicate memantine's benefits in severely demented patients.

Mild cognitive impairment. A memory impairment similar to that observed in mild Alzheimer's disease, but not great enough to interfere with a person's ability to live independently. People with this condition have about a 15 percent chance of developing Alzheimer's disease each year.

Milligram (mg). A measurement used for drugs equivalent to 1/1000 of a gram.

Nerve growth factor. A group of chemicals secreted by genetically engineered nerve cells, which stimulate neuron growth and boost the brain's cholinergic neurotransmitter system. A limitation of human use is the difficulty of getting nerve growth factor into the brain.

Neurofibrillary tangles. Collections of decayed material resulting from brain cell death and degeneration, present in high concentrations in the areas involved in memory in the Alzheimer's brain.

Neurogenesis. New nerve cell growth.

Neuron. Nerve or brain cell.

Neuropsychological tests. Standardized tests that measure memory, attention, and other cognitive abilities.

Neurotransmitter. A small molecule that serves as a brain messenger, allowing one neuron to communicate with another.

N-methyl-D-aspartate (NMDA) receptor antagonists. Drugs that work on the brain's NMDA receptors by blocking the brain chemical glutamate, which overstimulates these receptors, leading to cell destruction. The drug Namenda, which involves this mechanism, has been found to benefit patients with moderate to severe Alzheimer's disease.

Nonsteroidal anti-inflammatory drugs (NSAIDs). Drugs that interfere with the body's inflammatory process, generally used to treat minor injuries and arthritis. Examples include aspirin, ibuprofen (Motrin, Advil, Feldene), and cox-II inhibitors (Celebrex, Vioxx).

Nootropics. A class of drugs, including piracetam, oxiracetam, pramiracetam, and aniracetam, that enhances brain circulation. An anti-dementia effect has not been established, and controlled studies have yielded mixed results.

Nutraceutical. Natural substances not regulated by the FDA and used as supplements, often to counteract the aging process.

Objective memory ability. An individual's memory ability measured by standardized memory tests or neuropsychological tests.

Omega-3 fatty acids. So-called good fats that keep brain cell membranes soft and flexible and come from fruits, leafy vegetables, nuts, fish, and supplements.

Omega-6 fatty acids. So-called bad fats that tend to make brain cell membranes more rigid and come from animal meat, whole milk, cheese, margarine, mayonnaise, processed foods, fried foods, and vegetable oils.

Oxidative stress. The wear and tear that free radicals cause to the body's cells through a chemical reaction in which oxygen reacts with another substance to cause a chemical transformation. Antioxidants counteract this process.

Oxygen radical absorbency capacity (ORAC). The unit for a laboratory measuring technique that determines the ability of different foods to counteract oxidative stress. Foods with high ORAC scores may protect brain cells from the damage of oxygen radicals or free radicals.

Parietal lobe. The area of the brain above and behind the temporal region (near the temples), which controls some aspects of memory and cognition and is affected early in the course of Alzheimer's disease.

Pharmacogenetics. The emerging field of drug effectiveness and safety based upon an individual's genetic makeup.

Phosphatidylserine. A nutrient present in fish, green leafy vegetables, soy products, and rice, which some experts recommend as a supplement for age-associated memory impairment. Results of placebo-controlled studies have been positive but long-term benefits are not known. The recommended starting dose ranges from 200 to 300 mg daily followed by a maintenance dose of 100 mg daily after several months.

Physostigmine. A cholinesterase inhibitor drug with a very brief duration of action, such that the pills need to be taken every few hours for a memory effect. Although some studies demonstrate a mild benefit, it is not generally used and long-term effects are not known.

Positron emission tomography (PET). A body scanning method that measures structure as well as function. PET scans of the brain show characteristic patterns of decreased metabolism in the areas affected by Alzheimer's disease.

Protein. A molecule that is the building block of neurotransmitters and enzymes.

Rivastigmine (Exelon). A cholinesterase inhibitor drug used to treat Alzheimer's disease. Rivastigmine can be increased every two weeks beginning at 1.5 mg twice daily up to 6 mg twice daily or the highest dose tolerated. Dose increases should be slower if patients have difficulties tolerating side effects.

Selective estrogen receptor modulators (SERMs). New synthetic estrogens designed to isolate beneficial hormone effects and eliminate side effects. Studies have not yet shown SERMs to benefit cognitive function, but many experts remain optimistic of their eventual utility.

Selegiline (Eldepryl). A drug that inhibits monoamine oxidase enzymes that destroy neurotransmitters and has an antioxidant effect. Selegiline has been found to delay functional decline in patients with Alzheimer's disease. Because this effect is similar to that of vitamin E, and selegiline is more expensive and has more side effects, vitamin E is the preferred antioxidant treatment for Alzheimer's disease.

Serotonin. A neurotransmitter necessary for relaxation, concentration, and sleep that is decreased in depression and dementia.

Short-term memory. Memories lasting only minutes and too transient for long-term recall.

Smart drugs. Medications, herbs, hormones, or supplements taken with the intent of improving memory and other cognitive functions in a normal individual who does not have obvious memory loss.

Statins. Cholesterol-lowering drugs that may reduce the risk for developing Alzheimer's disease.

Stress response. The body's physiological reaction to stress, involving release of cortisol and other stress hormones.

Stroke. Death of brain cells resulting in a loss of physical or mental function or both.

Subdural hematomas. Blood clots surrounding the brain; a potential side effect of ginkgo biloba.

Subjective memory ability. A person's self-awareness of memory ability.

Synapse. The interface between two nerve cells where they communicate information.

Tacrine (Cognex). The first cholinesterase inhibitor approved by the FDA. The drug is rarely used today because of liver side effects and its frequent dosing schedule.

Testosterone. In men with low testosterone levels, the hormone may improve memory performance, and it is currently under investigation as a treatment for cognitive impairment.

Transcranial magnetic stimulation (TMS). An innovative noninvasive technique that uses head-mounted wire coils that produce powerful yet brief magnetic pulses directed at specific brain regions to cause brain cell firing in order to improve brain health. Initial studies suggest that TMS transiently improves memory performance, either during the procedure or shortly thereafter.

Vascular dementia. A dementia resulting from many small strokes.

Verbal memory. Learning and recall of information relating to language and words.

Vinpocetine. A dietary supplement that enhances brain circulation and has antioxidant properties. Several but not all studies demonstrate significant improvements in memory measures.

Visual-spatial memory. Learning and recall of visual and spatial information.

Vitamin C. An antioxidant vitamin that may offer protection against age-related cognitive decline. Many experts recommend 500 to 1,000 mg daily to slow age-related cognitive decline.

Vitamin E. An antioxidant vitamin prescribed in high doses (1,000 to 2,000 units daily) for patients with Alzheimer's disease. Epidemiological studies suggest that taking vitamin E supplements may slow age-related cognitive decline, and many experts recommend from 400 to 800 units daily as a preventive therapy.

Appendix 7:

Additional Resources

Many organizations provide information on memory and general health issues important to maintaining brain health. Several national organizations also have local or state chapters. Check your telephone directory or Internet search engine for related organizations and Web sites.

Name & Address	Description	Telephone
AARP 6601 E Street N.W. Washington, DC 20049 www.aarp.org	Nonprofit, nonpartisan organization dedicated to helping older Americans achieve lives of independence, dignity, and purpose.	202-434-2277 800-424-3410

Name & Address	Description	Telephone
Academy of Molecular Imaging Box 951735 Los Angeles, CA 90095-1735 www.ami-imaging.org	Provides leadership in research and clinical aspects of molecular imaging of the biological nature of disease. Their Web site includes a listing of local PET centers.	310-267-2614
Administration on Aging 330 Independence Avenue N.W. Washington, DC 20201 www.aoa.dhhs.gov	Provides information for older Americans and their families on opportunities and services to enrich their lives and support their independence.	202-619-7501 800-677-1116
Aging Network Services 4400 E. West Highway, Ste 907 Bethesda, MD 20814 www.agingnets.com	Nationwide network of private-practice geriatric social workers serving as care managers for seniors living at a distance.	301-657-4329
Alliance of Information and Referral Systems P.O. Box 31668 Seattle, WA 98103 www.airs.org	Professional organization that provides human services information and referrals.	206-632-2477

Name & Address	Description	Telephone
Alzheimer Europe 145 Route de Thionville L-2611 Luxembourg www.alzheimer-europe.org	Organizes caregiver support and raises awareness about dementia through cooperation among European Alzheimer's organizations.	352-29-79-70
Alzheimer's Association 919 N. Michigan Avenue, Ste 1000 Chicago, IL 60611-1676 www.alz.org	National organization that provides information on services, programs, publications, and local chapters.	800-272-3900
Alzheimer's Association Public Policy Division 1319 F Street N.W, Ste 710 Washington, DC 20004 www.alz.org	Lobbying branch of the Alzheimer's Association.	202-393-7737
Alzheimer's Foundation of America 252 W. 37th Street, 8th floor New York, NY 10018 www.alzfdn.org	National nonprofit foundation supporting organizations that help lighten the burden and improve the quality of life of Alzheimer's patients and their caregivers.	866-789-5423

Name & Address	Description	Telephone
Alzheimer's Disease Education & Referral Center P.O. Box 8250 Silver Spring, MD 20907 www.alzheimers.org	National Institute on Aging service that distributes information and free materials on topics relevant to health professionals, patients and their families, and the general public.	301-495-3311 800-438-4380
Alzheimer Research Forum 82 Devonshire Street, S3 Boston, MA 02109 www.alzforum.org	Provides information and promotes collaboration among researchers in order to foster a global effort to understand and treat Alzheimer's disease	
American Academy of Neurology 1080 Montreal Avenue St. Paul, MN 55116 www.aan.com	Professional organization that advances the art and science of neurology, thereby promoting the best possible care for patients with neurological disorders.	651-695-1940

Name & Address	Description	Telephone
American Association for Geriatric Psychiatry 7910 Woodmont Avenue #1050 Bethesda, MD 20814 www.aagpgpa.org	Professional organization dedicated to enhancing the mental health and well-being of older adults through education and research.	301-654-7850
American Diabetes Association P.O. Box 25757 1660 Duke Street Alexandria, VA 22314 www.diabetes.org	Nonprofit health organization providing diabetes research, information, and advocacy.	703-549-1500 800-232-3472
American Dietetic Association 216 W. Jackson Blvd. Chicago, IL 60606-6995 www.eatright.org	Consumer Nutrition Hotline that provides information on finding a dietitian.	312-899-0040 800-366-1655
American Geriatrics Society 770 Lexington Avenue #300 New York, NY 10021 www.americangeriatrics.org	Professional association providing assistance in identifying local geriatric physician referrals.	212-308-1414 800-247-4779

Name & Address	Description	Telephone
American Heart Association 7272 Greenville Avenue Dallas, TX 75231 www.americanheart.org	Nonprofit health organization whose mission is to reduce disability and death from cardiovascular diseases and stroke.	214-373-6300
American Society on Aging 833 Market Street, Ste 511 San Francisco, CA 94103 www.asaging.org	National organization concerned with physical, emotional, social, economic, and spiritual aspects of aging.	415-974-9600 800-537-9728
Children of Aging Parents 1609 Woodbourne Road, #302-A Levittown, PA 19057 www.caps4caregivers.org	National organization providing information and referrals for caregivers of older adults.	215-945-6900 800-227-7294
Family Caregiver Alliance 425 Bush Street, Ste 500 San Francisco, CA 94108 www.caregiver.org	Resource center for families of adults with brain damage or dementia, which provides publications for caregivers and professionals.	415-434-3388 800-445-8106

Name & Address	Description	Telephone
Gerontological Society of America 1030 15th Street N.W. Ste 250 Washington, DC 20005 www.geron.org	National interdisciplinary organization on research and education in aging.	202-842-1275
Memory Fitness Institute 24331 Muirlands Blvd. #D4-309 Lake Forest, CA 92630 www.memoryfitnessinstitute.org	The Memory Fitness Institute helps people of all ages to optimize their memory function and brain health, using state-of-the-art diagnostic, intervention, and prevention strategies.	866-7-memory
National Institute of Mental Health 5600 Fishers Lane, Room 10-75 Rockville, MD 20857 www.nimh.nih.gov	Part of the National Institutes of Health, the principal biomedical and behavioral research agency of the United States government.	301-443-1185

Name & Address	Description	Telephone
National Institute of Neurological Disorders and Stroke Building 31, Room 8A-06 31 Center Drive, MSC 2540 Bethesda, MD 20892-2540 www.ninds.nih.gov	The National Institutes of Health agency that supports neuroscience research; focuses on rapidly translating scientific discoveries into prevention, treatment, and cures; and provides resource support and information.	301-496-5751 800-352-9424
National Institute on Aging Building 31, Room 5C27 31 Center Drive Bethesda, MD 20892-2292 www.nih.gov/nia	The National Institutes of Health agency that supports research on aging and provides information about national Alzheimer's centers, and a free directory of organizations that serve older adults.	301-496-1752 800-438-4380
National Stroke Association 96 Inverness Drive East, Ste 1 Englewood, CO 80112-5112 www.stroke.org	Their mission is to reduce the incidence and impact of stroke disease and improve quality of patient care and outcomes.	303-649-9299 800-787-6537

Name & Address	Description	Telephone
Older Women's League 666 11th Street N.W. Ste 700 Washington, DC 20001 www.owl-national.org	An advocacy organiz-ation addressing family and caregiver issues.	202-783-6686 800-825-3695
Safe Return P.O. Box 9307 St. Louis, MO 63117-0307 www.alz.org	Joint program of the Alzheimer's Association and the National Center for Missing Persons that provides patients with a dementia bracelet show-ing the person's name, the registered caregiver's name, and a toll-free number (800-572-1122) to aid in that person's re-turn if lost.	888-572-8566
SeniorNet 121 Second Street, 7th Floor San Francisco, CA 94105 www.seniornet.org	A national nonprofit or-ganization that works to build a community of computer-using seniors.	415-495-4990

Name & Address	Description	Telephone
UCLA Center on Aging 10945 Le Conte Avenue #3119 Los Angeles, CA 90095-6980 www.aging.ucla.edu	University center that works to enhance and extend productive and healthy life through research and education on aging.	310-794-0676
U.S. Dept. of Veterans Affairs 1120 Vermont Avenue N.W. Washington, DC 20421 www.va.gov	Provides information on VA programs, veterans benefits, VA facilities worldwide, and VA medical automation software.	800-827-1000

Bibliography

Anthony GA, Grayson DA, Creasey HM, et al. Anti-inflammatory drugs protect against Alzheimer disease at low doses. *Arch Neurol* 2000;57:1586–91.

Appel LJ, Champagne CM, Harsha DW, et al. Effects of comprehensive lifestyle modification on blood pressure control: main results of the PREMIER clinical trial. *JAMA* 2003;289:2083–93.

Argyriou A, Prast H, Philippu A. Melatonin facilitates short-term memory. *Eur J Pharm* 1998;349:159–62.

Astin JA, Shapiro SL, Eisenberg DM, Forys KL. Mind-body medicine: state of the science, implications for practice. *J Am Board Fam Pract* 2003;16:131–47.

Balestreri R, Fontana L, Astengo F. A double-blind placebo controlled evaluation of the safety and efficacy of vinpocetine in the treatment of patients with chronic vascular senile cerebral dysfunction. *J Am Geriatr Soc* 1987;35:425–30.

Bai DL, Tang XC, He XC. Huperzine A, a potential therapeutic agent for treatment of Alzheimer's disease. *Curr Med Chem* 2000;7:355–74.

Ball K, Berch DB, Helmers KF, et al. Effects of cognitive training interventions with older adults: A randomized controlled trial. *JAMA* 2002;288:2271–81.

Barberger-Gateau P, Letenneur L, Deschamps V, et al. Fish, meat, and risk of dementia: cohort study. *Br Med J* 2002;395:932–33.

Benson H. *The Relaxation Response.* Avon, New York, 1975.

Bissoli L, Di Francesco V, Ballarin A, et al. Effect of vegetarian diet on homocysteine levels. *Ann Nutr Metab* 2002;46:73–9.

Blumenthal JA, Babyak M, Wei J, et al. Usefulness of psychosocial treatment of mental stress-induced myocardial ischemia in men. *Am J Cardiol* 2002;89: 164–8.

Bookheimer SY, Strojwas MH, Cohen MS, et al. Brain activation in people at genetic risk for Alzheimer's disease. *N Engl J Med* 2000;343:450–6.

Bowman RE, Beck KD, Luine VN. Chronic stress effects on memory: Sex differences in performance and monoaminergic activity. *Horm Behav* 2003; 43:48–59.

Brand-Miller J, Volwever TMS, Colaguiri S, Foster-Powell K. *The Glucose Revolution*. Marlow & Co, New York, 1999.

Brooks JO, Friedman L, Yesavage JA. Use of an external mnemonic to augment the efficacy of an internal mnemonic in older adults. *Int'l Psychogeriatr* 2003;15:59–67.

Calle EE, Rodriguez C, Walker-Thurmond K, Thun MJ. Overweight, obesity, and mortality from cancer in a prospectively studied cohort of U.S. adults. *N Engl J Med* 2003;348:1625–38.

Carper J. *Your Miracle Brain*. HarperCollins, New York, 2000.

Chainani-Wu N. Safety and anti-inflammatory activity of curcumin: a component of turmeric (Curcuma longa). *J Altern Complement Med* 2003;9: 161–8.

Colcombe SJ, Erickson KI, Raz N, et al. Aerobic fitness reduces brain tissue loss in aging humans. *J Gerontol: Med Sci* 2003;58A:176–80.

Collins MW, Grindel SH, Lovell MR, et al. Relationship between concussion and neuropsychological performance in college football players. *JAMA* 1999; 282;964–70.

Convit A, Wolf OT, Tarshish C, de Leon MJ. Reduced glucose tolerance is associated with poor memory performance and hippocampal atrophy among normal elderly. *Proc Natl Acad Sci USA* 2003;100:2019–22.

Cook NR, Albert MS, Berkman LF, et al. Interrelationships of peak expiratory flow rate with physical and cognitive function in the elderly: MacArthur Foundation studies of aging. *J Gerontol A Biol Sci Med Sci* 1995;50:M317–23.

Crisby M, Carlson LA, Winblad B. Statins in the prevention and treatment of Alzheimer disease. *Alzheimer Dis Assoc Disord* 2002;16:131–6.

Del Ser T, Hachinski V, Merskey H, Munoz DG. An autopsy-verified study of the effect of education on degenerative dementia. *Brain* 1999;122:2309–19.

De Smet PAGM. Herbal remedies. *N Engl J Med* 2002;347:2046–56.

Devanand DP. *The Memory Program*. John Wiley & Sons, New York, 2001.

Dickey RA, Janick JJ. Lifestyle modifications in the prevention and treatment of hypertension. *Public Health Nutr* 1999;2:383–90.

Edwards P, Lhotsky M, Turner J. *The Healthy Boomer: A No-Nonsense Midlife Health Guide for Women and Men.* McClelland & Stewart Inc, Toronto, 1999.

Ehlenfeldt MK, Prior RL. Oxygen Radical Absorbance Capacity (ORAC) and phenolic and anthocyanin concentrations in fruit and leaf tissues of highbush blueberry. *J Agric Food Chem* 2001;49:2222–7.

Eng PM, Fitzmaurice G, Kubzansky LD, Rimm EB, Kawachi I. Anger expression and risk of stroke and coronary heart disease among male health professionals. *Psychosom Med* 2003;65:100–10.

Engelhart MJ, Geerlings MI, Ruitenberg A, et al. Dietary intake of antioxidants and risk of Alzheimer disease. *JAMA* 2002;287:3223–9.

Ercoli LM, Small GW, Silverman DHS, et al. The effects of ginkgo biloba on cognitive and cerebral metabolic function in age-associated memory impairment. Society for Neuroscience Abstract, 2003.

Eriksson J, Lindstrom J, Tuomilehto J. Potential for the prevention of type 2 diabetes. *Br Med Bull* 2001;60:183–99.

Ernst ND, Sempos ST, Briefel RR, Clark MB. Consistency between US dietary fat intake and serum total cholesterol concentrations: the National Health and Nutrition Examination surveys. *Am J Clin Nutr* 1997;66:965S–2S.

Fairfield KM, Fletcher RH. Vitamins for chronic disease prevention in adults: scientific review. *JAMA* 2002;287:3116–26.

Fetrow CW, Avila JR. *The Complete Guide to Herbal Medicines.* Pocket Books, New York, 2000.

Fillit HM, Butler RN, O'Connell AW, et al. Achieving and maintaining cognitive vitality with aging. *Mayo Clin Proc* 2002;77:681–96.

Foster GD, Wyatt HR, Hill JO, et al. A randomized trial of a low-carbohydrate diet for obesity. *N Engl J Med* 2003;348:2082–90.

Friedland RP, Fritsch T, Smyth KA, et al. Patients with Alzheimer's disease have reduced activities in midlife compared with healthy control-group members. *Proc Natl Acad Sci USA* 2001;98:3440–5.

Frishman WH. Are antihypertensive agents protective against dementia? A review of clinical and preclinical data. *Heart Dis* 2002;4:380–6.

Gage FH. Neurogenesis in the adult brain. *J Neurosci* 2002;22:612–3.

Gilewski MJ, Zelinski EM, Schaie KW. The Memory Functioning Questionnaire for assessment of memory complaints in adulthood and old age. *Psychology and Aging* 1990;5:482–90.

Golier JA, Yehuda R, Lupien SJ, Harvey PD, Grossman R, Elokin A. Memory performance in Holocaust survivors with posttraumatic stress disorder. *Am J Psychiatry* 2002;159:1682–8.

Grandjean AC, Reimers KJ, Bannick KE, Haven MC. The effect of caffeinated, non-caffeinated, caloric and non-caloric beverages on hydration. *J Am Coll Nutr* 2000;19:591–600.

Green CS, Bavelier D. Action video game modifies visual selective attention. *Nature* 2003;423:534–7.

Gustafson D, Rothenberg E, Blennow K, Steen B, Skoog I. An 18-year follow-up of overweight and risk of Alzheimer disease. *Arch Int Med* 2003;163:1524–8.

Haier RJ, Siegel BV, MacLachlan A, et al. Regional glucose metabolic changes after learning a complex visuospatial/motor task: A positron emission tomographic study. *Brain Research* 1992;570:134–43.

Hathcock JN. Vitamins and minerals: Efficacy and safety. *Am J Clin Nutr* 1997;66:427–37.

He FJ, MacGregor GA. Effect of modest salt reduction on blood pressure: a meta-analysis of randomized trials. Implications for public health. *J Hum Hypertens* 2002;16:761–70.

Heber D, Bowerman S. *What Color Is Your Diet?* ReganBooks, New York, 2001.

Hebert LE, Scherr PA, Bienias JL, Bennett DA, Evans DA. Alzheimer disease in the US population: prevalence estimates using the 2000 census. *Arch Neurol* 2003;60:1119–22.

High KP. Micronutrient supplementation and immune function in the elderly. *CID* 1999;28:717–22.

Hightower JM, Moore D. Mercury levels in high-end consumers of fish. *Environ Health Perspect* 2003;111:604–8.

Hui KK, Liu J, Makris N, et al. Acupuncture modulates the limbic system and subcortical gray structures of the human brain: evidence from MRI studies in normal subjects. *Hum Brain Mapp* 2000;9:13–25.

Irwin MR, Pike JL, Cole JC, Oxman MN. Effects of a behavioral intervention, tai chi chih, on varicella-zoster virus specific immunity and health functioning in older adults. *Psychosom Med* 2003;65:824–30.

Jick H, Zornberg GL, Jick SS, et al. Statins and the risk of dementia. *Lancet* 2000;356:1627–31.

Joseph JA, Nadeau D, Underwood A. *The Color Code: A Revolutionary Eating Plan for Optimum Health*. Hyperion, New York, 2002.

Kahn RL, Rowe JW. *Successful Aging*. Pantheon, New York, 1998.

Keefer L, Blanchard EB. A one year follow-up of relaxation response meditation as a treatment for irritable bowel syndrome. *Behav Res Ther* 2002;40:541–6.

Kidd PM. A review of nutrients and botanicals in the integrative management of cognitive dysfunction. *Altern Med Rev* 1999;4:144–61.

Kleijnen J, Knipschild P. Ginkgo biloba. *Lancet* 1992;340:1136–40.

Kramer AF, Hahn S, Cohen NJ, et al. Ageing, fitness and neurocognitive function. *Nature* 1999;400:418–9.

Kramer AF, Hahn S, McAuley E, et al. Exercise, aging and cognition: Healthy body, healthy mind? In Fisk AD, Rogers W (eds). *Human Factors Interventions for the Health Care of Older Adults*. Erlbaum, Hillsdale, NJ, 2001.

Larsson CL, Johansson GK. Dietary intake and nutritional status of young vegans and omnivores in Sweden. *Am J Clin Nutr* 2002;76:100–6.

Lazar JS. Mind-body medicine in primary care. Implications and applications. *Prim Care* 1996;23:169–82.

Lazar SW, Bush G, Gollub RL, et al. Functional brain mapping of the relaxation response and meditation. *Neuroreport* 2000;11:1581–5.

Lindsay J, Laurin D, Verreault R, et al. Risk factors for Alzheimer's disease: a prospective analysis from the Canadian Study of Health and Aging. *Am J Epidemiol* 2002;156:445–53.

Lorayne H. *How to Develop a Super Power Memory*. Lifetime Books, Hollywood, FL, 1998.

Ma Y, Bertone ER, Stanek EJ 3rd, et al. Association between eating patterns and obesity in a free-living US adult population. *Am J Epidemiol* 2003;158:85–92.

Matser JT, Kessels AG, Lezak MD, Jordan BD, Troost J. Neuropsychological impairment in amateur soccer players. *JAMA* 1999;282:971–3.

Mattson MP. Existing data suggest that Alzheimer's disease is preventable. *Ann NY Acad Sci* 2000;924:153–9.

McEwen B. *The End of Stress As We Know It*. The Dana Press, Joseph Henry Press, Washington, DC, 2002.

Merchant C, Tang MX, Albert S, et al. The influence of smoking on the risk of Alzheimer's disease. *Neurology* 1999;52:1408–12.

Middlekauff HR, Hui K, Yu JL, et al. Acupuncture inhibits sympathetic activation during mental stress in advanced heart failure patients. *J Card Fail* 2002;8:399–406.

Miller JJ, Fletcher K, Kabat-Zinn J. Three-year follow-up and clinical implications of a mindfulness meditation-based stress reduction intervention in the treatment of anxiety disorders. *Gen Hosp Psychiatry* 1995;17:192–200.

Montgomery SA, Thal LJ, Amrein R. Meta-analysis of double blind randomized controlled clinical trials of acetyl-L-carnitine versus placebo in the treatment of mild cognitive impairment and mild Alzheimer's disease. *Int Clin Psychopharm* 2003;18:61–71.

Morris MC, Beckett LA, Scherr PA, et al. Vitamin E and vitamin C supplement use and risk of incident Alzheimer disease. *Alzheim Dis Assoc Disord* 1998;12:121–6.

Mukamal KJ, Kuller LH, Fitzpatrick AL, et al. Prospective study of alcohol consumption and risk of dementia in older adults. *JAMA* 2003;289:1405–13.

National Center for Health Statistics. Healthy people 2000 review, 1997. Hyattsville, Maryland: US Department of Health and Human Services, CDC, 1997.

Natural Medicines Comprehensive Database. www.naturaldatabase.com.

Newcomer JW, Selke G, Melson AK, et al. Decreased memory performance in healthy humans induced by stress-level cortisol treatment. *Arch Gen Psychiatry* 1999;56:527–33.

Newman PE. Could diet be used to reduce the risk of Alzheimer's disease? *Medical Hypotheses* 1998;50:335–7.

Paivio A, Yuille JC, Madigan SA. Concreteness, imagery, and meaningfulness values for 925 nouns. *J Exp Psych Monograph Suppl* 1968;76:1–25.

Polich J, Gloria R. Cognitive effects of a ginkgo biloba/vinpocetine compound in normal adults: systematic assessment of perception, attention and memory. *Hum Psychopharmacol Clin Exp* 2001;16:409–16.

Raskind MA, Peskind ER, Wessel T, and the Galantamine USA-1 Study Group. Galantamine in AD: A 6-month randomized, placebo-controlled trial with a 6-month extension. *Neurology* 2000;54:2269–76.

Reisberg B, Doody R, Stoffler A, et al. Memantine in moderate-to-severe Alzheimer's disease. *N Engl J Med* 2003;348:1333–41.

Rennie MJ. Claims for the anabolic effects of growth hormone: a case of the Emperor's new clothes? *Br J Sports Med* 2003;37:100–5.

Ritchie K. Mental status examination of an exceptional case of longevity: J. C. aged 118 years. *Br J Psychiatry* 1995;166:229–35.

Rubinstein JS, Meyer DE, Evans JE. Executive control of cognitive processes in task switching. *J Exp Psychol Hum Percept Perform* 2001;27:763–97.

Ruitenberg A, van Swieten JC, Witteman JC, et al. Alcohol consumption and risk of dementia: the Rotterdam Study. *Lancet* 2002;359:281–6.

Sapolsky RM. Glucocorticoids, stress, and their adverse neurological effects: relevance to aging. *Exp Gerontol* 1999;34:721–32.

Satoh T, Sakurai I, Mihagi K, Hohsaku Y. Walking exercise and improved neuropsychological functioning in elderly patients with cardiac disease. *J Internal Med* 1995;238:423–8.

Scarmeas N, Levy G, Tang MX, Manly J, Stern Y. Influence of leisure activity on the incidence of Alzheimer's disease. *Neurology* 2001;57:2236–42.

Shapiro D, Jamner LD, Goldstein IR, Delfino RJ. Striking a chord: moods, blood pressure, and heart rate in everyday life. *Psychophysiology* 2001;38:197–204.

Shoghi-Jadid K, Small GW, Agdeppa ED, et al. Localization of neurofibrillary tangles and beta-amyloid plaques in the brains of living patients with Alzheimer disease. *Am J Geriatr Psychiatry* 2002;10:24–35.

Shumaker SA, Legault C, Rapp SR, et al. Estrogen plus progestin and the incidence of dementia and mild cognitive impairment in postmenopausal women. The Women's Health Initiative Memory Study: a randomized controlled trial. *JAMA* 2003;289:2651–62.

Silverberg GD, Levinthal E, Sullivan EV, et al. Assessment of low-flow CSF drainage as a treatment for AD: results of a randomized pilot study. *Neurology* 2002;59:1139–45.

Skolnick AA. Old Chinese herbal medicine used for fever yields possible new Alzheimer disease therapy. *JAMA* 1997;277:776.

Small G. *The Memory Bible: An Innovative Strategy for Keeping Your Brain Young.* Hyperion, New York, 2002.

Small GW. What we need to know about age related memory loss. *Br Med J* 2002;324:1502–5.

Small GW, Ercoli LM, Silverman DHS, et al. Cerebral metabolic and cognitive decline in persons at genetic risk for Alzheimer's disease. *Proc Natl Acad Sciences USA* 2000;97:6037–42.

Solfrizzi V, Panza F, Torres F, Mastroianni F, Del Parigi A, Venezia A, Capurso A. High monounsaturated fatty acids intake protects against age-related cognitive decline. *Neurology* 1999;52:1563–9.

Spencer JW, Jacobs JJ (Eds). *Complementary/Alternative Medicine: An Evidence-Based Approach.* Mosby-Year Book, St. Louis, 1999.

Stern Y. The concept of cognitive reserve: a catalyst for research. *J Clin Exp Neuropsychol* 2003;25:589–93.

Taylor-Piliae RE. Tai chi as an adjunct to cardiac rehabilitation exercise training. *J Cardiopulm Rehab* 2003;23:90–6.

Trichopoulou A, Costacou T, Bamia C, Trichopoulos D. Adherence to a Mediterranean diet and survival in a Greek population. *N Engl J Med* 2003;348:2599–608.

van Boxtel MP, Paas FG, Houx PJ, et al. Aerobic capacity and cognitive performance in a cross-sectional aging study. *Med Sci Sports Exercise* 1997; 29:1357–65.

Van Dongen HPA, Maislin G, Mullington JM, Dinges DF. The cumulative cost of additional wakefulness: Dose-response effects on neurobehavioral functions and sleep physiology from chronic sleep restriction and total sleep deprivation. *Sleep* 2003;2:117–26.

Van Praag H, Kempermann G, Gage FH. Neural consequences of environmental enrichment. *Nat Rev Neurosci* 2000;1:191–8.

Vance ML. Can growth hormone prevent aging? *N Engl J Med* 2003; 348:779–80.

Verghese J, Lipton RB, Katz MJ, et al. Leisure activities and the risk of dementia in the elderly. *N Engl J Med* 2003;348:2508–16.

Wallis C. Guess what F is for? Fat. *Time* Sept. 15, 2003, pp. 68–9.

Wansink B, Linder LR. Interactions between forms of fat consumption and restaurant bread consumption. *Int J Obesity* 2003;27:866–8.

Yesavage JA, Mumenthaler MS, Taylor JL, et al. Donepezil and flight simulator performance: effects on retention of complex skills. *Neurology* 2002; 59:123–5.

Zelinski EM, Gilewski MJ, Anthony-Bergstone CR. Memory Functioning Questionnaire: concurrent validity with memory performance and self-reported memory failures. *Psychology and Aging* 1990;5:388–99.

Zollman C, Vickers A. ABC of complementary medicine: What is complementary medicine? *Br Med J* 1999;319:693–6.

Permissions and Source Credits

Chapter 2

Subjective Memory Questionnaire adapted with permission from the work of Dr. Michael Gilewski (Gilewski et al. 1990).

Chapter 3

Photographs by Rena Small. Models (in order of appearance): Andy Garb, Cynthia Bougoukalos, Dr. Shirley Impellizzeri, Amy Gandin, Rachel Small, Valerie Grant, and Dr. Max Small.

Frozen banana/peanut-butter sandwich with permission from Hermien Lee.

Chapter 6

Photographs by Rena Small. Models (in order of appearance): Amy Gandin, Sheila Garb, Stuart Grant, and Cynthia Bougoukalos.

Chapter 9

Photographs by Rena Small. Models (in order of appearance): Dr. Shirley Impellizzeri, Amy Gandin, Cynthia Bougoukalos, and Dr. Tom Marinaro.

Appendix 4

PET scans showing brain function patterns courtesy of Michael Phelps, Ph.D., UCLA Department of Molecular and Medical Pharmacology.

Graph showing six-month delay in cholinergic treatment adapted from Raskind et al. 2000.

Index

ability to learn
    multitasking and, 204
    stress and, 194
acetyl-l-carnitine, 261
acetylcholine, 256, 261, 263, 264
acronyms, 148
active observation, 142
active observation exercises, 143
acupressure, 208
acupuncture, 208–9
adrenaline, 191, 194
aerobic conditioning, 16, 108, 110
    tailoring, 27
    see also physical aerobic conditioning
aerobic exercise/aerobics, 214, 224
    and cardiac health, 197
    stimulates production of endorphins,
    218
aerobic exercise component
    with diet, 30
aerobic workout breaks, 222–23
African Americans, 166
age
    brain shrinks with, 216, 217
    and chronic illness, 248
    and memory challenges, 1–2
    and objective memory score, 23
age-related condition(s), inheriting, 5

aging, 256
    and brain cell damage, 165
    dangerous effects of, 249
    muscle loss in, 227
    premature, 195
    protection from effects of, 5, 17–18, 245
    and side effects of medications, 254
aging process
    slow, stop, reverse, 33
alcohol, 34, 249
    protecting brain, 176–77
allostatic load, 190–91, 192
aluminum, 184–85
Alzheimer's disease, 2, 8, 23, 167, 247, 253,
    298–314
    amyloid plaques, 251
    and anti-inflammatory drugs, 252
    antioxidants and, 267
    delaying, 286
    dietary supplements and, 261–62, 264
    drugs in treatment of, 255, 257
    hormones and, 259
    intellectual activity and, 115
    leisure activity and, 198
    overweight and, 164–65
    physical activity and, 216
    prevalence of, 10–11
    vitamin B_{12} for, 266

Index

Alzheimer's disease, risk for, 27, 170
    aerobic conditioning and, 215
    aluminum and, 184
    head injury and, 229
    mental activity and, 114
    statins and, 250
Alzheimer's risk gene, 9, 10, 229
amino acids, 259, 263
amitriptyline (Elavil), 253
ampakines, 258
amyloid plaques, 8, 229, 250, 251, 256
anger, expressing, 196–97
anger management, 199, 209
anger management techniques, 14
anger modulation, 196, 197
anti-Alzheimer's drugs
    who should take, 255–58
anticholinergic side effects, 254
antidepressant/antianxiety medications, 210,
    252–53
anti-inflammatory drugs, 251–52
antioxidant movement, 266–67
antioxidant-rich foods, 161, 162
antioxidant supplements, 34, 162, 267
antioxidants, 170, 171, 172
anxiety, 23, 24, 196, 200, 214, 218
    controlling, 187
    drugs for, 254–55
    psychotherapy for, 210
apolipoprotein E-4 (APOE-4), 9, 10, 229
appetite, 179
    controlling, 162–63, 167–68
arginine, 259
Arkansas, 163
arthritis, 195
Ashtanga, 203
aspirin, 251, 252
assessment tests, 16
atherosclerosis, 181
Atkins, Dr., 167
Atkins Diet, 166, 167
atorvastatin (Lipitor), 250
attention, focused, 142, 205

ß-carotene, 266
back pain, 208, 228
balance, 217, 226, 228
baseline scores, 1
    comparing "after" assessment results with,
    103

    objective memory, 105
    subjective memory ability, 18, 21
baselines
    charting, for setting goals, 31–32
    physical stamina status, 16
    stress level, 25
Bextra, 252
Big 4, 4, 11, 273–74, 282
    managing, 33
    physical fitness in, 214
    scientific findings supporting, 112
bingeing
    bad for brain, 162–65
biofeedback, 206
blood-brain barrier, 255
blood pressure, 6
    controlling, 249
    emotions and, 196
    lowering, with diet, 180
    see also high blood pressure (hypertension)
blood sugar
    crashes, 187
    foods causing spikes in, 173, 175–76
    and memory loss, 173–74
blood sugar level(s), 172, 173, 174
blowing off steam
    to protect brain, 196–97
BMI (body mass index), 163
    and dementia/Alzheimer's disease, 164–65
body
    keeping young for life, 285–86
body weight
    see weight
brain
    alcohol protecting, 176–77
    bingeing bad for, 162–65
    blowing off steam to protect, 196–97
    boot camp for, 11–12
    cross training, 117
    fats and, 165–68
    front part of, 204
    keeping young for life, 285–86
    left hemisphere, 17
    protecting, 6, 7, 8–11
    right hemisphere, 17
    shrinks with age, 216, 217
    sugar for, 172–76
brain aging, 6–7, 8, 9
    aerobic conditioning and, 215
    chronic stress in, 190

diet in, 161
head injury and, 229
homocysteine and, 182
oxidative stress in, 169
staving off, 11
stress and, 195
brain and body health, strategies for, 11
brain bingeing, 164
brain/body connection, 215
brain boosters
    cholinesterase inhibitors as, 256–57
brain cells, 10, 165
    damage/death, 6, 165, 251, 266
    development and regeneration, 167
    growing, 115–16
    new, 216
    protection of, 252
    sleep and connection between, 200
    "stretching and toning" workout, 114
brain circulation, 167, 226, 230, 263
brain efficiency, 6, 9–10
    adding to, with external aids, 270–73
    improved, 13
brain fitness, 10
    dietary supplements and, 265
    foods that help or hinder, 188–89
    physical activity in, 226
    physical fitness and, 245
    protecting, 254
    sleep deprivation in, 200–1
    threats to, 255
brain food alternatives, 188–89
brain function, 14
brain health
    maintaining, 282
    physical fitness and, 215
    pumping iron for, 226–27
brain hemisphere(s), 17, 117, 118, 119
brain imaging technologies, 11
brain power
    hormones for, 258–65
brain-protective effects of aerobic conditioning,
        215–17
brain regions
    and memory, 140
brain safety, 229–30
brain stress test, 9, 13, 146
brainpower, building, 118
brainteasers, 114, 123, 137
breakfast, 178

breaks, taking, 210–11
breathing techniques, 199
building bulk, 179

caffeine, 185–87, 261
caffeine intoxication, 186
caffeine withdrawal, 186
calcium, 182
calendars, 271
calories, 6, 162
    empty, 163–64
cancer, 162, 165, 169, 195, 267
cancer drugs, 255
carbo load, 172
carbohydrates, 162, 167, 172–73
card games
    winning at, 156–69
cardiac patients, 14
cardiovascular disease, 195
    risk for, 167
cardiovascular fitness
    and brain shrinkage, 216
cardiovascular problems, stress in,
        190
cataracts, 169
Celebrex, 252
chemo brain, 255
Chi Gong, 203
children
    and mercury toxicity, 168
    overweight, 163
chill out, 212
cholesterol, 6, 167, 214
    caffeine and, 185
    high, 31, 181–82
    high: risk for, 166
    managing, 181–82
cholesterol-lowering statins, 249–50
cholinergic drugs, 256
cholinergic system, 253, 262
cholinesterase inhibitors
    as brain boosters, 256–57
chronic back pain, 208
chronic brain inflammation, 167
chronic fatigue syndrome, 190
chronic illness, 248
chronic insomnia, 200, 201
chronic stress, 4, 24, 26, 192
    and brain aging, 190
    and immune system, 195

chronic stress syndrome, 192
chunking information, 151, 156
    exercises for, 153–55
cigarette smoking, 6, 7
clioquiniline, 258
coenzyme Q_{10}, 261–62
cognition
    aspirin and, 252
cognitive approach to stress reduction, 199
cognitive decline/impairment, 253
    antioxidants and, 267
    drugs in treatment of, 258
    hypertension and, 248
    preventing, 257
    with sleep deprivation, 200
    see also mild cognitive impairment
cognitive function, 263
cognitive reserve, 115
cognitive training, 140
concentration, 265
    difficulties with, in depression, 252
concussion, 229
confidence, 16–17, 103–4
CONNECT (linking mental snapshots),
    145–49
    see also LOOK, SNAP, CONNECT
connecting exercises, 147, 148–49
coordination, 226, 228
corn oil, 166
coronary artery disease, 181
    stress management and, 197–98
corticosterone, 195
cortisol, 195, 249
counting and mathematics, 117
cox-II inhibitors, 252
creatine, 262
cross-training, 117, 220, 223–24
crossword puzzles, 113–14
curcumin, 262
cyclooxygenase II, 252

daily planning lists, 271
daily progress reports
    worksheets for, 296–97
daily routines, 273
dancing, 225
date books, 272
delegating, 194
dementia, 10, 163, 253
    alcohol and, 176–77

and anti-inflammatory drugs, 252
BMI and, 164–65
caffeine and, 185
cholinesterase inhibiors in treatment of, 257
delaying onset of, 256
dietary supplements and, 262, 263, 264
drugs in treatment of, 257, 258
homocysteine and, 182
hormones and, 258, 259
late-stage, 10
mental activity and risk for, 114–15
risk for, 8, 166, 196, 198, 225
dementia with Lewy bodies, 257
depression, 195, 196, 214, 218
    anger and, 197
    psychotherapy for, 210
    sleep and, 200, 201
    treatment for, 252–53
DHEA (dehydroepiandrosterone), 258
diabetes, 31, 167, 173, 182, 195, 214, 217, 248,
    267
    blood sugar problems and, 174
    risk for, 13–14, 163, 166
    stress and, 190
diet, 5, 111, 273
    bad, fatty, 2
    high protein/low carbohydrate, 166–67
    see also 14–Day Memory Prescription Diet
diet, healthy, 2, 14, 248
    with physical exercise, 13–14
diet, healthy brain, 11, 14, 16, 33, 34, 108, 187,
    222
diet tips, 183–89
dietary needs, assessing, 45
Dietary Supplement Health and Education Act,
    260
dietary supplements, 260–65
    see also supplements; vitamin supplements
dimethylaminoethanol (DMAE), 262
distress, 211
dl-phenylalanine, 263
DNA, 169
docosahexaenic acid (DHA), 264
doctor(s)
    checking medications, 263
    consulting, 23, 26, 28, 29, 35, 178, 179, 201,
        225, 229, 248, 250, 255, 259, 267
donepezil (Aricept), 256, 257
drug addiction, 164
drug interactions, 254–55, 260, 263

drugs, 247–68
    anti-Alzheimer, 255–58
    anti-inflammatory, 251–52
    for hypertension, 248–49
    keeping brain young with, 268
    memory-enhancing, 258

eating, healthy, 4
eating habits, 163
education/educational level
    and Alzheimer's disease, 115
    and brain activity, 10
    brain-protective effects of, 115
    and objective memory score, 23
effort, 116
elastic exercise band, 230
electronic hand-held organizers, 272
emotions, dealing with, 196–97
empowerment, feeling of, 103–4
endorphins, 202, 208, 214, 263
    aerobic exercise and, 218
energy (chi), 209
essential amino acids, 263
estrogen, 249, 258, 259
exaggeration, 144
executive control center, 204, 217
exercise
    and brain cell growth, 216
    healthy diet with, 13–14
    finding right workout, 224–26
    getting high on, 217–18
    see also aerobic exercise/aerobics; physical
        activity; physical conditioning
exercise duration, 222, 224
exercise program, 214
    customizing, 223
expectations, unreasonable, 210
external memory tools, 270–73
    worksheets, 273–81

faces
    connecting names to, 151
    remembering, 145, 149–52
famous person or place
    names associated with, 150
fatigue, 200
fats
    and the brain, 165–68
    good/bad, 165–66
fibromyalgia, 208

"fight or flight" response, 191
fish, 166, 167
    mercury in, 168–69
    substitutions for, 179–80
fish oil supplements, 167
fitness gadgets, 227–28
fitness level(s)
    see mental fitness level; physical fitness level
five meals a day, 178
fluoxetine (Prozac), 253
fluvastatin (Lescol), 250
focus, 203, 204
    on details, 144
    on an object, 205
focusing attention, 142, 205
folate/folic acid, 266
food, 161, 177
    mental effects of, 187
food substitutions, 34
    in day-by-day plan, 101–2
foods
    effect on brain fitness, 188–89
    fat-free, 165
    in managing cholesterol, 181–82
    spiking blood sugar, 175–76
14–Day Memory Prescription, 2, 4, 5–6, 11, 17,
        21, 31, 33–102, 139, 140, 149, 199, 209
    adjusting, 25, 34
    aerobic conditioning, 110
    aerobic workout breaks, 222–23
    augmenting, 137
    augmenting physical fitness component of, 230
    balance in, 222
    completing, 103, 111–15
    CONNECT exercises in, 146
    daily supplement regimen, 248
    day-by-day plan, 35–102
    "Fitness on the Run" segments, 223
    individualizing, 23
    memory skills/techniques, 23, 104, 140
    mental aerobics, 114, 118
    multivitamin supplement in, 254–55
    personalized, 4, 14
    physical fitness component, 27, 28, 224
    physical fitness pump-up, 223–24
    refilling for life, 14–15
    refining memory training component of, 108
    relaxation response in, 205
    renewing, 12, 30, 31, 112, 137, 269–86
    renewing: building tools for, 273–81

14–Day Memory Prescription (*continued*)
  renewing: how it's done, 282–85
  stress-release breaks in, 211
  stress release exercises, 26, 108
  stressing stress reduction in, 198–201
  tailoring to individual needs, 16, 103
  tips before beginning, 34–35
14–Day Memory Prescription Diet, 28–31, 111, 112, 161–89, 269
  goals in, 162
  grocery list, 287–89
  making work for you, 177–83
  modifications to, 28, 29
  omega-3 supplements in, 264
  recipes for, 290–95
14–Day Memory Prescription Diet worksheet, 276–77
free association, 148
free radicals, 169–70, 264, 266, 267
free weights, 227–28
frontal lobe, 141, 217
frontotemporal dementia, 257
fruits and vegetables, 164, 167, 174, 266
  antioxidant, 171, 172
fun, 118, 138, 212
fun factor, 116
functional MRI scans, 9, 115, 141, 198, 209
  brain test, 13

galantamine (Reminyl), 257
genetic risk, 5, 8, 10
ginkgo biloba, 261, 263
glucose, 263
  see also sugar
glutamate, 257
glycemic index, 162, 173, 174, 175, 187
glycogen, 172–73
green tea, 172
grocery list, 287–89
growth hormone stimulants, 259
guided imagery, 199

habits, 6
  healthy, 269, 274
  lifestyle, 66
  lifestyle changes becoming, 12
  lifetime, 285
  memory, 272
  of mental aerobics, 116
  quality longevity, 14

head injuries, 229–30
health
  stretching and toning for better, 230–45
heart attack
  anger and, 196
  risk for, 185, 216
  risk for death from, 249
heart disease, 6, 162, 182
  protection from, 166, 266
  risk for, 165, 180, 196
  see also cardiovascular disease
herbal remedies, 260–61
high blood pressure (hypertension), 31, 214, 217, 248
  caffeine and, 185
  diet and, 180
  drugs for, 248–49
  risk for, 163, 166
high protein/low carbohydrate diets, 166–67
hippocampus, 115–16, 140–41, 164, 174, 204
  chronic stress and, 195
  new cells in, 216
  size of, 117
hobby(ies), 137
homocysteine, 182
hormones, 161, 204, 249
  for brain power, 258–65
huperzine a, 263–64
hydergine, 258
hypertension
  see high blood pressure (hypertension)

ibuprofen (Motrin, Advil, Nuprin), 251, 252
illnesses
  medicines for, 253–54
imipramine (Tofranil), 253
immune function, 266
immune system
  stress and, 190, 195
indomethacin (Indocin), 251
infection risks, 265–66
inflammation, 161, 165, 167, 251, 252
  in brain, 166
  minimizing, 264
information
  arranging, 152–54
  attributing meaning to, 141, 144
  transforming into visual images, 144

information sequencing, 117
information storage, 140
injuries, 218, 219–22, 223, 225, 227
    head, 229–30
    lowering risk for, 230
insomnia, 200, 201
    beating, 201–2
insulin, 167, 173, 261
insulin resistance, 167, 173
insulin spikes, 174, 187
interleukin-6 (IL-6), 195
internal memory tools, 270
International Olympic Committee, 258
Internet, 119
intervention, focused, 11
Inuit Eskimos, 166
Iyengar, 203

jogging, 199, 225, 226
Journal of the American Medical Association,
    140, 176

ketotic state, 167
kicking back, 209–12
knees, 228–29
Kripalu, 203

language and speech, 117
LDL cholesterol, 181, 249
learning, 21, 140, 141, 145, 270
lecithin, 264
left-brain exercises
    see mental aerobics exercises
left-brain functions, 117
leisure activities, 211–12
    involving mental effort, 225
    and risk for Alzheimer's disease, 198
Librium, 255
lifestyle, 33
    exercise in, 223
    healthy, 182
    mentally taxing, 118
    and sleep problems, 199–200
lifesyle changes, 12
    with hypertension, 249
    to protect brain, 11
    and risk for high cholesterol, 249
lifestyle choices, 5, 8
lifestyle habits, new, 66
link method, 147–48, 156

lipoic acid, 261
liquids, 183–84
logical analysis, 117
long-term memory, 140–41, 144, 218
longevity, 7
    eating for, 161–89
    healthy, 15
    medicine's role in, 247
    see also quality longevity
longevity program, 33
LOOK (active observation), 65, 142
    see also LOOK, SNAP, CONNECT
LOOK, SNAP, CONNECT, 35, 48–49, 54, 56,
    63–64, 67–68, 69, 70–71, 76–77, 90, 93,
    94, 156, 160, 270
    remembering names and faces, 150–52
lovastatin (Mevacor), 250
low glycemic-index carbohydrates, 162, 174,
    175
lycopene, 172

magnetic resonance imaging (MRI), 9, 174
    see also functional MRI scans
massage, 199, 208
meaning
    attributing to information, 141, 144
medications/medicines
    antidepressant/antianxiety, 210, 252–53
    drug interactions, 254–55
    for high blood pressure, 180
    new, 247–48
    for other illnesses, 253–54
medicine, modern
    role in longevity, 247
meditation, 198, 199, 205, 211
Mediterranean Diet, 162, 166
melatonin, 264
memantine (Namenda), 257
memory
    antioxidants and, 267
    dietary supplements and, 264, 265
    effect of stress on, 4, 194–95
    effects of physical aerobic conditioning on,
        216–17
    hormones and, 259, 260
    improvement in, 6
    insomnia and, 200
    long-term/short-term, 140–41, 144, 218
    mood and, 217–18
    multivitamins and, 266

Index

memory (*continued*)
  omega-6 fatty acids and, 167
  stretching and toning for better, 230–45
memory ability, 270
  antioxidants and, 170
  assessing, 4, 17–18
memory aids, choosing, 272
memory challenges in aging, 1–2
memory changes, worry about, 23
memory decline, 11
  protection against future, 286
  statins preventing, 250
memory-enhancing drugs, 258
memory fitness, 266–67
  maintaining, 282
memory fitness movement, 7
memory fitness program/strategies, 6, 9–10, 17
memory function
  back pain and, 228
  dancing and, 225
memory habits, 272
memory impairments
  in athletes, 229–30
  from drugs, 255
Memory International meeting, 139
memory load
  organization to reduce, 152–54
memory loss, 163
  anger and, 196
  blood sugar problems and, 174
  dietary supplements and, 261–62, 263, 264
  drugs in treatment of, 257
  hormones in treatment of, 258
  inflammation in, 251
  preventing, 254
memory performance
  aerobic conditioning and, 215
  improved, 13, 16
memory places, 271
memory power
  expanding, 154–56
Memory Prescription Study, 13–14
memory pro, becoming, 154–56
memory slips
  in depression, 252–53
memory techniques/skills, 35, 118, 145, 154
  fine-tuning, 140
  learning, 139
  LOOK, SNAP, CONNECT, 141–54

  meaning in, 141
  taking to next level, 156–59
  training in, 23
memory training, 2, 23, 112
  advanced, 16, 139–60
memory training exercises, 20–21
memory training techniques
  advanced, 270
  building blocks for, 149
men
  ideal body weight, 30
mental activity, 4, 10, 11, 33, 222, 274
  earlier in life, 115
  and risk for Alzheimer's disease, 114
mental activity worksheet, 278–79
mental aerobic exercises, 34–35, 118–37, 199
  advanced exercises, 131–37
  beginning exercises, 119–23
  intermediate exercises, 123–31
  varying, 223–24
mental aerobics, 112
  high-impact, 114–16
  individualizing, 118
  pumping up, 113–38
  right level of, 113, 123
  see also under 14–Day Memory Prescription, day-by-day plan
mental aerobics program, building, 137–38
mental attention, 217
mental conditioning, 14
mental decline, 7
  intellectual activity and, 114
  see also cognitive decline/impairment
mental effort, 198
  leisure activities involving, 225
mental fitness level
  rating, 16–32
mental inactivity, 2
mental performance
  effects of physical aerobic conditioning on, 216–17
mental snapshot exercises, 145
mental snapshots, creating, 143–44
mental stimulation, 198
mentally taxing jobs, 118
mercury, 168–69
meridians, 209
methyl mercury, 168
Metropolitan Life Insurance Company, 29

mild cognitive impairment, 256, 257
  hormones and, 259
mind
  aerobicizing, 118–37
mixed dementias, 257
mnemonic method, 156, 270
moderation, 218, 219
mood
  dietary supplements and, 264
  hormones and, 259, 260
  improvement in, 6, 16
  and memory, 217–18
  sleep and, 200
multitasking, 8, 140, 194
  saying no to, 203–4
multivitamins, 34, 248, 267
muscle mass, loss of, 226–27
myotherapy, 208

names
  categories of, 150
  connecting to faces, 151
  remembering, 145, 149–52
naproxyn (Aleve), 251, 252
naps, 201, 211
National Cancer Institute, 164
National Center for Complementary and
    Alternative Medicine, 261
National Football League, 258
Natural Medicines Comprehensive Database, 261
natural products, 258, 259, 261
neurofibrillary tangles, 8
neurogenesis, 10, 115–16
neuropsychological testing, 21
neurotransmitters, 263
niacin, 266
Nigerians, 166
nitric oxide, 250
NMDA receptor antagonist, 257
"no pain no gain" mantra, 218–19
nonsteroidal anti-inflammatory drugs
    (NSAIDs), 251
notes, effective, 271
nucleus accumbens, 164
numbers
  method to memorize, 156–59

obesity, 163, 165, 173
  physical illnesses related to, 217
  risk for, 178, 179

objective memory abilities, 16
  assessing, 21–23
  reassessing, 103
Objective Memory Assessment No. 1, 22–23
Objective Memory Assessment No. 2, 104–5
objective memory assessment score, 17
  updating, 104–5
objective memory performance baseline, 31
objective memory scores
  interpreting, 24
  reviewing, 119
O'Brien, Dominic, 139
olive oil, 166, 168
omega-3 fatty acids, 34, 162, 165, 166, 167–68,
    169, 181
  sources other than fish, 179–80
omega-3 supplements, 248, 264–65
omega-6 fatty acids, 161, 162, 166–67, 179
organization
  to reduce memory load, 152–54
organizational skills, 153, 270
osteoporosis, 185, 195
overweight, 163, 178
  and Alzheimer's disease, 164–65
  see also obesity
oxidation, 161, 266
oxidative stress, 164, 169–70
oxygen radical absorbency capacity (ORAC),
    170

pancreas, 173
Parkinson's disease, 185, 267
paroxetine (Paxil), 253
Peg Method, 156–59
perspective, putting things in, 210
PET scan
  see positron emission tomography (PET
    scanning)
phone numbers, 153, 156
phosphatidylserine, 265
photographic memory, 139, 154
physical activity(ies), 4, 226
  cardiac patients, 14
  length of, 222–23
  in stress reduction, 199
physical aerobic conditioning, 112
  protecting brain cells, 252
  to release stress, 202
  and sex, 214–15
  see also aerobic conditioning

Index

physical conditioning, 2, 4, 5, 10, 11, 13, 33, 35,
    222, 248, 274
  and brain health, 27
  makes us feel good, 218
  reassessing status, 103
physical conditioning worksheet, 280–81
physical fitness, 14
  baseline, 31, 32
  and brain fitness, 245
  and brain health, 215
physical fitness activity, 179
physical fitness conditioning
  finding right workout, 224–26
physical fitness jump-start, 214–46
physical fitness level
  assessing, 27–28
  rating, 16–32
  reassessing, 110–11
physical fitness pump-up, 223–24
Physical Fitness Questionnaire, 27–28, 110–11,
    215
physician(s)
  see doctor(s)
physiological responses, controlling, 206
physostigmine, 258
Pilates, 199, 226, 228
Pilates, Joseph, 226
pineal gland, 264
piroxicam (Feldene), 251
placebo effect, 13
playfulness, 144
portion sizes, 34, 179
positron emission tomography (PET scanning),
    8, 9–10, 13, 17
  in diagnosing Alzheimer's, 255–56
post-hypnotic suggestions, 205
Post-its, 272
post-traumatic stress disorder, 195
power nap, 201, 211
"powerhouse," 226, 228
pravastatin (Pravachol), 250
prefrontal cortex, 140
prevention/preventive treatment, 6–7, 11, 252
Proceedings of the National Academy of
    Sciences, 174
progestin, 259
progress
  visuals in charting, 281–82
progressive muscle relaxation techniques,
    197, 209

prostate cancer, 260
protein, 162
  sources of, 182
pseudodementia, 253
psychological variables
  in diet, 164
psychotherapy, 199, 209–10
pumping iron, 226–27
pumping up, 215–17
puzzles, 114, 115, 123, 137

quality longevity, 2, 4, 14, 18, 218
  enemy of, 24
  lifetime of, 269–86
quality of life, 247, 260

racquet sports, 225
reading and writing, 117
recall, 21, 23, 140, 141, 144, 145, 270
  multitasking and, 204
  stress and, 194, 195
recipes, 34, 290–95
relaxation exercises, 206–8
relaxation response, 199, 202
  paths to, 204–8
relaxation techniques, 198
research update, 315–23
riboflavin, 182, 266
right-brain exercises
  see mental aerobics exercises
right-brain functions, 117
rivastigmine (Exelon), 256, 257
Roman Room Method, 154–56, 158
runner's high, 218

sadness, 197, 252, 253
salt, 180
seasonal affective disorder, 218
selenium, 182
self-awareness
  of improvement, 16–17
  of memory loss, 17, 21
self-hypnosis, 199, 205
senses, using, 142
serotonin, 198, 209, 264
sertraline (Zoloft), 253
sex
  physical aerobic conditioning and, 214–15
shopping for food, 34
short-term memory, 218

side effects, 254–55
  antidepressants, 253
  anti-inflammatory drugs, 252
  cholinesterase inhibitors, 256
  DHEA, 258
  growth hormone stimulants, 259
  mental, 255
  statins, 250
  simvastatin (Zocor), 250
sleep, 199–202
sleep deprivation, 199–201
sleep hygiene, 35
sleep inducement
  systematic approach to, 201–2
smoking
  quitting, 249
SNAP (creating mental snapshots), 95, 143–45,
    151, 158
  and CONNECT, 63–64, 69, 87, 88, 94
  methods of connecting, 146
  real/imagined, 144
  see also LOOK, SNAP, CONNECT
statins, 249–50
story system, 147–48
strengthening, 228
strengthening exercises, 239–44
stress, 2, 5, 214
  effects of, 194–95
  internally driven, 210
  minimizing, 212–13
  subliminal, 194
  see also chronic stress
stress eating
  cutting out, 187–88
stress energy, 202
stress hormones, 191, 192, 196
  depression and, 253
  and memory loss, 194, 195
Stress Level Questionnaire, 25–26, 109–10, 199
stress levels, 16
  assessing, 4
  baseline, 31, 32
  reassessing, 103, 108–10
stress-management instruction, 197–98
stress reduction, 2, 4, 10, 11, 13, 14, 23, 33,
    112, 190–213, 272, 273
  cardiac patients, 14
  physical activity in, 226
  through relaxation response, 204–5
  stressing, 198–201

stress reduction exercise, 123
stress reduction techniques, 16, 248
Stress Reduction Worksheet, 274–75
stress-release breaks, 211
  see also under 14–Day Memory Prescription,
    day-by-day plan
stress release, 198
  physical aerobic conditioning in, 202
stress-release activities, 26, 108, 209
  physical/mental components, 202–3
stress responses, 190–94, 204
stressed out, 24–26, 190
stretching, 35, 223, 224, 228
  for better health and memory, 230–45
stretching exercises, 231–39
stroke(s), 6, 163, 173, 180, 181, 217
  alcohol and, 177
  defined, 248–49
  protection from, 266
  risk for, 167, 196, 216, 250
subjective memory abilities, 16
  assessing, 105–8
  rating, 17, 18–21, 23
  reassessing, 103
subjective memory performance baseline, 31
subjective memory questionnaire, 18–20, 106–8
subjective memory scores
  interpreting, 24
  reviewing, 119
success
  gauging, 103–12
sugar
  for brain, 172–76
supplements, 247–68
  keeping brain young with, 268
Swedish massage, 208
swimming, 223, 225
symbol recognition, 117
synergy, 13–14
  between physical stress reduction and
    conditioning, 199

tacrine (Cognex), 256
tai chi, 199, 203
"talk test," 218
taste
  and craving, 164
tennis, 225
testosterone, 258, 260
Thai massage, 208

thiamine, 266
toning, 224, 228
    for better health and memory, 230–45
trans-fatty acids, 165
treadmills, 227–28
treatments, 11, 208–9
trigger points, 208
triglycerides, 181
2–week checkup, 103–12

UCLA Neuropsychiatric Institute, 203
UCLA research, 6, 8, 9, 11, 16, 17, 31, 103,
    162, 245
    Memory Prescription Study, 13–14
unwinding, 209–12
urinary bladder cancer, 185
U.S. Environmental Protection Agency (EPA),
    168, 169
U.S. Food and Drug Administration, 169, 256,
    258, 259

Valium, 255
vascular dementia, 257
vegetarians, 182–83
    alternative sources of basic nutrients for,
    183
vinpocetine, 265
Vioxx, 252
visual image
    names evoking, 150–51
visuals
    to chart progress, 281–82
vitamin A, 266
Vitamin B$_{12}$, 182, 266
vitamin C, 34, 170, 266
    antioxidant, 267
    supplement, 248
vitamin D, 182, 266
vitamin E, 34, 170, 266
    antioxidant, 267
    supplement, 248

vitamin K, 266
vitamin supplements, 34, 170, 265–66
    antioxidant, 267
    see also supplements

walking/walks, 199, 216, 217, 224, 226
warm-up/cool-down routine(s), 224, 230
water, 183–84
weighing in
    on day 14, 111
weight
    baseline, 31, 32
    controlling, 214, 217
    ideal, 28–30, 178, 179
    pads of, 161
weight gain, 164
weight loss, 34, 103, 110
    liquids and, 184
    Memory Prescription Diet in, 178–79
    omega-3 fatty acids in, 167–68
weight machines, 227–28
weight reduction program, 30
weight training, 217, 227
well-being, sense of, 108, 205, 210
women
    ideal body weights, 29
work, 211–12
working memory, 140, 141
working out, 214
worksheets, 273–81
    for daily progress reports, 296–97
    Memory Prescription Diet, 276–77
    mental activity, 278–79
    physical conditioning, 280–81
    stress reduction, 274–75
World Memory Championship, 139
writing things down, 270, 271

Xanax, 255

Yoga, 199, 202–3, 211